Every Mile Matters

Compiled by Moon Joggers

DEDICATION

To every runner, walker and jogger out there.

ACKNOWLEDGMENTS

A group of runners, walkers and joggers from around the world have taken the time to share what EVERY MILE MATTERS means to them. Each person shares their own stories and how running and walking has impacted their lives. Every Mile Matters no matter how fast or how slow you go.

Every Mile Matters
by Amanda Duffin

"You really went out this morning and ran?' asked my father-in-law slightly skeptical.

The snowfall flitted outside the window of the diner where we were having coffee. His raised eyebrow told me he was hesitant to believe me, but the tilt of his head told me he did not know me to be a practical joker.

"Yes," I said with a chuckle. "I really ran. I did a 10k this morning,"

"Really." he said, now resigned to believe me. "How far is that?"

How far is that? What an interesting question. I suppose the easy answer is 6.2 miles, but it's not true. Like taking a photograph during a trip, that day's run captured only a moment of a much larger journey.

The truth is, it took me 558 miles to get to those 6.2 that I called a 10k. And all of it, every step, good and bad, mattered.

I decided to take up running in the summer of 2013. I had a few friends who had started running. I had walked a few 5ks in previous years, but it never occurred to me to try to run. Apparently, it had occurred to them. They were off and I was amazed.

In June 2013, I put my then one-year-old in her lightweight, flip and click stroller, laced up my beat up sneakers and went for a walk to the local bike trail.

It was bad.

I went 2.75 miles. It took me nearly an hour. And when I was done, I thought about giving up the whole idea. I felt exhausted for the rest of the day. When I woke up the next morning my body felt sluggish and heavy.

It made me doubt myself and I wanted to quit. But I had a baby to take care of, and she would grow into a child that wanted to play. Would I be able to play?

We went out again.

I kept at it even though I felt awful afterwards. Every other day we went for a walk and, gradually, the heaviness started to lift. Gradually, I realized I could go for a walk and not wake up worn out the next morning.

It was noticeable, tangible progress. And it was encouraging.

We started to walk everyday, even on weekends. We started to go farther, faster. And one day in the fall, I decided it was time to jog instead of walk.

It was bad.

The stroller was wrong. The shoes were wrong. My clothes were wrong. Everything was wrong. My lungs burned. My head throbbed. My back ached. And that voice said, "What the hell were you thinking? You can't do this."

Fortunately, I learned one of my friends who used to walk 5ks was training for a marathon. A marathon! She wasn't born running. She trained. She worked. She didn't give up.

When I started, walking a couple of miles was exhausting, but now it was no sweat. I had improved with work. She worked for her marathon and got there. My dream was smaller. I wanted to run a 5k. If I worked, surely, I could get there too.

I went to a real running store and bought real running shoes. I hit the yard sales and found a jogging stroller in good shape. I scoured the clearance racks and turned up some steals on running clothes. I put together a running playlist. I read. I asked questions. I found Moon Joggers.

By spring 2014, I was not only better prepared, I was chomping at the bit to get outside. I started the Couch to 5k program. I signed up for virtual runs to motivate myself. I adjusted my exercise schedule as my daughter's routine changed. Instead of turning around half way through, I started running program sessions completely before turning back to come home, even if I walked the whole way back.

It was good.

I did 52 miles in March, a personal best. By July, I shattered it, logging 108 miles and running my best 5k to date – 34:01. In September, the opportunity to do a 10k came. I was coming off injury, but I did it. In November, I did it again and better.

Not only could I tell my physical health was improving. I found I felt less stress. I felt happier. I was proud of my body, not because I lost weight, but because I learned my body was capable of amazing things. And in all aspects of my life, I found improved confidence.

I traveled 558 miles, on an amazing journey, to get to that November finish line.

Sipping coffee in the diner, I thought about telling my father-in-law all this. But in the end, I just gave the simple answer.

   "A 10k is 6.2 miles," I said. "It's a long 6.2 miles"

About the author:
Amanda Duffin lives in Alhambra, Il. with her husband and 2 year old daughter. She currently works in public relations at an advertising agency. In her spare time, you can find Amanda running, cooking and doing science experiments with her toddler.

Every Mile Matters
by Jaclynn Williams

When I volunteered to write one of these articles a couple of months ago, I figured that someone with my running background would safely secure a spot later in the year...October or November, maybe. I can't say I was especially excited to see my name on the list for mid-January. I struggled with what to write...what on earth could someone like me have to contribute? For a few days, I seriously considered asking to have my name removed completely. But, after a decent run and a pep talk from my loving husband (something about how it takes all kinds, I think), I didn't. And now, here I am, trying to put into words what the phrase "Every Mile Matters" means to me.

A dear friend of mine was in a biking accident this summer. He suffered temporary paralysis and has been undergoing extensive physical therapy, as well as speech therapy. He's doing well, but it has been heartbreaking to watch someone I love deal with the pain and extreme frustration of a traumatic brain injury. A few weeks ago, we walked two miles together, humming Christmas songs and looking at decorated houses. A few months ago, he couldn't move his legs...and he walked with me. I will treasure those two miles for the rest of my life.

On Christmas day, after too many sweets and beers, I convinced my little brother to go for a run with me. He lives out of state and I rarely see him, so I was thrilled to have a little time to spend together, catching up. We planned to run two miles. Before leaving the house, he informed me that he had never run more than a 5K and hadn't run at all for quite some time. We had deep and insightful conversations, enjoyed an unseasonably lovely Kansas afternoon and, before we knew it, we had run more than 6 miles. We had such a great time, and I was so proud of him for more than doubling what he thought he was able to run. Another few miles that I will hold in my heart always.

Why does a mile matter to me? I'm not a competitive runner. I don't really aspire to be fast, and I enjoy beer and fried foods too much to be lean and fit. I enjoy running in events, but I often go months without signing up for any. Many days, I have no idea why I lace up my running shoes or slap on a "wicking base layer" and a fleece hat.

Life is hectic. Life is good, but it's certainly not perfect. Days are filled with errands, diapers, e-mails, dirty dishes, and a stressful, time-consuming job. Every mile I move is about 11 minutes of my life that I spend just moving. Just thinking and dreaming, all by myself. My running experience is VERY limited but even so, it's full of small moments that will always stay with me…memories that happened on the roads, not in front of a screen, in my bed, or sprawled out on the couch in pajamas.

I remember my cross-country running roommate dragging me out exactly once in college to run a mile. I remember having to stop about ¼ of the way in, and telling myself I would never attempt to run again. It was much too difficult, and it made my legs hurt. That was 14 years ago.

I remember when I tried to take up running when I lived in Arizona, and how I used to run while it was still dark before work. All I ever thought about, every single mile, was what I would do if a mountain lion suddenly appeared while I was running. When I left Arizona, I gave up on running completely….for almost a decade!

I remember the slow, painfully excruciating miles when I decided to give the running thing another try three years ago. It seems so long ago, but I still remember in detail the first time I was FINALLY able to make it a mile without stopping to walk.

I remember my first 5K. I was 12 weeks pregnant and was certain I wouldn't make it further than a mile...but I RAN that 5K. And then I ate two Big Macs and a large order of fries and spent three days sleeping on the couch.

I remember that mile last year, when I ran straight into a raised piece of sidewalk. I took the skin off both knees and could barely walk for a month. I considered giving up the whole running thing again...much too dangerous for someone as clumsy as me. As soon as my knees healed up a little, I signed up for another 5K and began looking for 10K runs.

I remember my first 10K run. I felt like I was moving SO slow, and it was SO cold...but I finished. I told myself I would never run farther than 10K...that would be insane.

I remember the first time I ran more than 8 miles. At mile 7, a random stranger in street clothes stopped me to give me tips about my foot strike. I'm STILL irritated with him.

I remember when a friend texted me recently, asking me if I would do a half marathon with her in the spring. I didn't respond to her text message for a few days...she had clearly lost her mind. Then, after a particularly good run, I responded. I texted "yes...let's find one!" The date...April 11...is now written on my calendar. I'm scared to death.

I remember when I ran my 300th mile of 2014. I was less than a tenth of a mile from being done, and was trying to sprint the last bit...but the director of the cemetery (yes...I love to run in the cemetery...it's the only place where I know I will be the fastest!) pulled up to talk to me and it ended up being one of my slowest miles ever. It was a little anticlimactic, considering that my goal for 2014 was to break 300 miles...but that seems to be how the runs I think will be earth-shattering end up.

I remember my last run of 2014. I planned to run 6 miles...but, at the 6-mile mark, I got my second wind. I decided I would just keep going. I ran 12 miles! Prior to that day, the longest I had run was about 9 miles. I was ecstatic…until I almost passed out. I didn't realize I was supposed to have a snack or something during a run that long. Lesson learned.

I remember one of my first runs of 2015. I was planning to take a few days off, due to the extremely cold temperatures. But, I had just received confirmation that I had been paired off with an awesome little boy through the "I Run 4 Siblings" program. There was no way I could skip a few days of running, so I bundled up and knocked out the three coldest miles I had ever done. When I got home, my little buddy sent me a message that I should drink some hot chocolate. I did.

I will never be on the cover of a running magazine. Realistically, I'll never break 1,000 miles in a year. I will never run a 7 minute mile. I will sometimes skip runs in favor of watching TV or taking a nap. But I'll collect those miles. I'll collect them, and I'll store them away in my heart. Because those miles represent stories. And our lives are made of stories…good or bad, boring or silly, motivating or discouraging. Each mile is an opportunity…an opportunity to inspire or support someone, an opportunity to experience failure or pain, an opportunity to overcome an obstacle, an opportunity to learn something, or an opportunity to take a positive step toward a goal. I'm proud of my miles, because they are part of me. I'm proud to be a part of a wonderful community in which everyone is valued and every accomplishment…no matter how tiny…is celebrated.

About Jaclynn:
I'm a 2nd grade teacher in Lawrence, KS. I'm also a wife and the mama of a sweet 2-year old boy and an 8-year old chocolate lab. I have run off and on, here and there, in little chunks, for over a decade. I only became serious about my desire to be a life-long runner last spring. When I'm not running I enjoy books, good beers, play dates with friends, my church, cooking, and drinking black coffee while in my pajamas.

Every Mile Matters
by Marie Smith

Every mile matters,
but it isn't just about how far you go.
The journey is an experience,
With each foot-fall you throw

Be it a run, jog or walk,
you've taken that step to go
Relish the sights and sounds,
You'd otherwise not get to know.

Sun rise, or sun-set,
In wind, rain or snow.
A mile is just a measure,
It's the experience that makes you grow.

Enjoy the music of your feet,
that hit upon the ground.
Discovering not only the hidden world around you,
but also that there is a little part of yourself to be found.

EVERY MILE MATTERS
by Perry Newburn

When I put my hand up to write this I thought "this should be straight forward," but the more I thought about it – yes dangerous this thinking lark – the harder it became. So where to start?

I've written about my battles with addiction in the past but this point really stands out. What was a huge factor in helping me overcome the " battle"? It was of course exercise. I started to run again, play sport, and generally started to crawl my way back into the land of living. I didn't realize it at the time – I certainly do now – but the effect any form of exercise has, in a positive way, on peoples mental wellness is huge. After a bad day at work, on the home front, if there is a chance to go for a walk, bike or run take it as a lot (well most) of the perceived problems just seem to fade away. I remember talking to a running mate once and he explained that on getting home after " 1 of those days " his wife wanted to sit down and catch up on the day. He stated he would like to go for a run first of which she agreed. On arriving back he stated he was in a much better frame of mind and thoroughly enjoyed the " togetherness" time.

Hence why I have a huge advocate for the positive effect that any form of exercise has on peoples mental wellness. On my run around NZ (5000 km in 70 days) where I was running for the Mental Health Foundation of NZ I also used the opportunity to advocate for this as much as possible. So yes miles do matter when it comes to people's mental wellness.
Let's fast forward in time to when I joined the Moon Joggers at the start of 2013. I had just come off my NZ run a couple of months prior and had set a goal of running around our Lake Taupo (a distance of 155 km's), not just once but twice so I needed to keep the mileage up with a balance between recovery and training – yes every mile matters. Also I had never kept a tally of how many miles/km's I ran each week so I also set a goal of running 100 miles per week for the year. The support of this group has been huge in helping me meet targets, set goals that are at least close to being achievable plus above all else – TO HAVE FUN. Just a point here – I believe setting goals are so important as

9

they are something to strive towards but at the end of the day if they are not reached (and there are often lots of reasons why) we learn from them and gain immensely in the process. So yes with setting goals and then looking at what sort of training is necessary every mile matters to help you get there.

At about this time I set the goal of Running Across America in the shortest time possible so again every mile that was gained in the training process (18 months and approximately 12000 miles) to help me achieve this mattered.

On arriving back from the states I found out that I had a nasty little virus and am on 24 weeks of a nasty combination of medications of which I am now about half way through. So for me, again, every mile matters and it pretty well reverts back to why I originally got back into running – yes my mental wellness. Initially I thought I would be lucky to get 2-300 miles per month but actually managed 425 miles in January- yes my stubbornness does help!!! My regime at present is: 6am – 8 km mainly walk which helps immensely in clearing the brain fogginess and tiredness out of the body; 1030am – approximately a 15 km mainly run. Weekends I am now managing a longer run of approximately 30 km's. So again every mile does matter as it is helping me keep a balance – mentally – on things. The beauty is – all going well – I will be back much stronger and with a lot more energy.

So everyone, keep enjoying your exercise, keep having fun and above all else look after yourselves.

YES EVERY MILE MATTERS.

EVERY MILE MATTERS
by Angie Webb

As a child I loved to run, but I hated running. Give me a basketball or soccer ball and I could run for hours. Tell me to go and run a mile and I wouldn't do it. In Junior High School I played on the basketball, soccer and softball teams. I dominated dodge ball and flag football in P.E. It was Wednesdays that I dreaded most: the day of the "FUN" run.

On Those days I did not want to dress down and wished I had the guts to cut class. I could not see the "FUN" in running a mile and a half. Why in the world would someone run when there was no one chasing you down the field to steal the ball from you or sprinting down the court to score a fast break layup? In my mind, the only purpose for running was when you were playing sports. That's it.

I reminded myself of this every Wednesday as I slowly got dressed into my P.E. clothes and sluggishly walked out to the track. My "FUN" run consisted of hanging out with the other girls at the back of the pack, complaining about having to do a stupid mile and a half, and trying to get away with as little running as possible. Needless to say, my "FUN" runs were usually more of a "FUN" walk, with a small bit of running whenever Coach Bitton blew her whistle and told us to get moving.

My high school days were not much different. I played varsity basketball and soccer, and to me, running was a punishment. It was something we had to do when someone missed a free throw in practice or when our soccer coach would get frustrated and send us off on a mile run. My teammates and I did whatever we could to get out of running in our strength and conditioning class, which was taught by Coach Morgan, the football coach. When he wasn't looking, we'd take turns hiding, or we'd bribe him with donuts to get out of running laps. Fortunately, the donuts usually did the trick.

It wasn't until I moved away to college that I decided to give this whole running thing a try. I went down to St. George with my parents to watch my mom run the St. George Marathon. It was the first time I'd ever witnessed anything like that. I stood in awe as I watched people, both young and old, run the final 300 yards of a 26.2 mile run and I was overcome with emotion. I cried as I watched a little boy run out and run the final 100 feet, hand in hand, with his mom. I clapped for the older man that came limping in, but determined to cross that finish line.

Then there was my mom, a 49-year-old mother of eight children, running the final stretch. I could see the pain in her face as she struggled towards the finish, but she smiled as she completed her marathon. In that moment I caught the bug. Or should I say, the bug caught me. It bit me so hard and all I could think about was crossing that finish line.

I moved back to my home state of Utah to finish my degree at the University of Utah. It was during this time that I fell in love with running. I registered for the St. George Marathon and when I found out that I got in then the serious training began. I had only run in one event before and it was a small 5K in Anchorage, Alaska. The thought of running 26.2 miles was overwhelming, but once again, the thought of crossing the finish line pushed me forward.

My second semester of college I signed up for a 6:00am running class. Don't ask me what I was thinking signing up for such an early class, but I did it and I never missed. I wish I could say I fell in love with running right from the start, but that would be a lie. It was hard. I wanted to quit. I wanted to walk, and a few times I did. An added bonus is that I attended my first few semesters of college in Hawaii and I loved running on the beach. My friend, Anjanelle, and I would go for a run and then jump in the ocean for a refreshing swim. During that time I caught small glimpses of how "FUN" running could be and how good it made me feel.

During one of my training runs I discovered the runner's high. It was a clear, sunny morning filled with bright blue sky. The trees lining the roads were covered in fresh snow that had fallen the night before. I took off for a five mile run through my sleepy little neighborhood. As I ran, water dripped onto the street as the snow started to melt from the branches and I felt so alive. I felt like I could run forever and I did not want to stop. My whole body felt awake, alert and so very strong. Whenever I ran I craved to have that feeling, and although it didn't always happen, I loved how good running made me feel – physically, mentally and emotionally.

Running the St. George Marathon was an amazing experience for me. My mom also ran it that year and it was fun to share the experience with the person that inspired me to do it in the first place. There were 7,000 runners and I loved being part of the crowd and the excitement at the starting line. For the first mile I listened as thousands of feet hit the pavement. I'll never forget that. I felt so connected as my own feet joined in the rumbling chorus.
I wish I could say that the run was easy. It was definitely one of the hardest things I've ever done and there were a couple of times I was ready to call it quits. The finish line seemed to be thousands of miles away. But I kept putting one foot in front of the other and eventually the end was in sight. With about 200 yards left I was slowly dragging my aching legs towards the finish line when an older man came to my side and said, "You're not going to let a 60 year old man beat you to the finish line are you?" He had a huge grin on his face and started running fast, nearly sprinting, as he pulled ahead of me. In that moment I forgot about the pain and I pulled every ounce of energy I had left, and began to sprint. I crossed that finish line neck and neck with that man and then he gave me a smile and was gone.

I had completed a marathon. My whole body was sore and my legs felt like jelly when I finished, but I did finish. That day I realized that I can do anything. My body is strong and my feet will carry my wherever I ask them to go. Later that day I lost a toenail and for two weeks my legs hurt so bad. Walking up stairs or sitting down on the toilet was excruciating, but it was all worth it. Soon enough my body healed and I was out running again. In the next few years I ran several half marathons and went through phases where I ran and where I didn't run. It was a beautiful love-hate relationship. And through it all I can see how important each and every mile is, especially those miles that carried me to the starting line of my first marathon.

Every Mile Matters
By Iva Haines

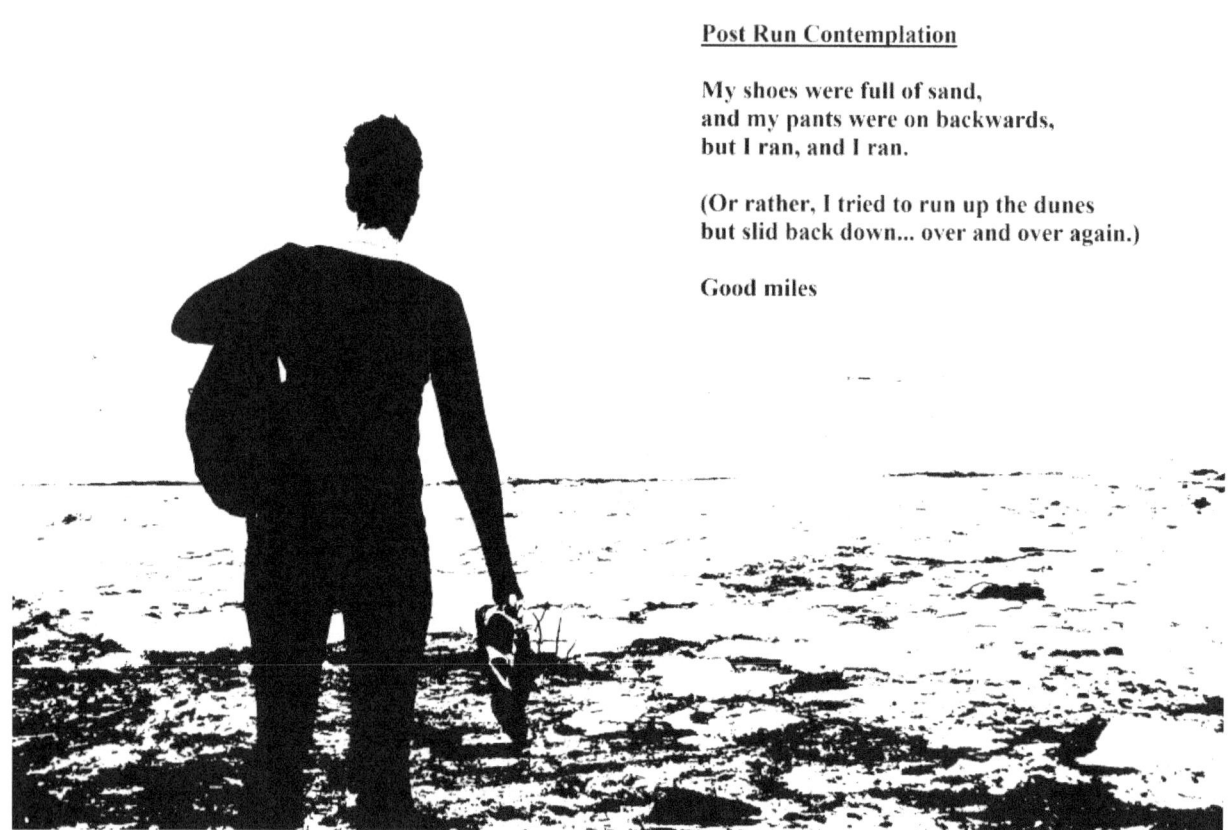

Post Run Contemplation

My shoes were full of sand,
and my pants were on backwards,
but I ran, and I ran.

(Or rather, I tried to run up the dunes
but slid back down... over and over again.)

Good miles

Why I Accomplished "Nothing" Today
(A stream of consciousness that came to me during my run)
by Maggie Hillis

A hiker visiting from Memphis fell off Signal Mountain to his death late last night/early this morning. That's really horrible, and I feel for his loved ones and hate that his life was cut so short and I hope those last few minutes were filled with awe and wonder and the same breathlessness I feel every time I stand in a spot very much like the one where he was when he fell, which is often.

That has absolutely nothing to do with why I failed to accomplish anything today on my endless list of things I have to do during this two weeks out of a cumulative 3 months I will spend at home this year.

It did, however, pass into my mind as I was planning my route for the day:

Riverside or mountain...
Flat and fast 10k on a paved route convenient to where I need to be later or whatever I can muster that will be at all more than what I did the other day on that mountain...
Rest my muscles or push myself harder...
Will there be a lot of people...
Do I crave the encouragement of other runners or the solitude of my own thoughts today in the on and off drizzle and falling leaves....
flowing water or falling leaves...
pavement or gravel....
I have a lot to do today, I really shouldn't go far...

I chose the wide flat slow climb up the mountain. It's not too far out of my way. It's a perfect, quite drizzly day for the mountain. And as I start out I think about how on this particular trail it would really take some effort to fall to one's death. I'm safe. I even left a note with a hand drawn map of my route on the kitchen table, and donned my running safety vest just in case. I always carry my phone.

Now, focus.

My form is good, I'm watching my step for unsteady ground and potential trip/ ankle twisting hazards. I perfect my breathing. I visually gage my half mile point in the distance, then mile one- focusing, pushing…this hurts a little, but in a good way, and I can keep going. No one's here. I am not in a race. I can stop and rest every half mile if I want. I can even walk some. This is *my* run. The important thing is that I finish. Finish what? I decide on 5 miles.
After a mile it gets harder, steeper, the terrain rougher, but the focus and the push slowly fade as I adjust, balancing heart rate, cadence, and breath till I don't realize I'm doing it. I slowly forget I'm doing anything at all….

Leaves whisper as the negligible breeze carries them earthward…
Autumn seems to have come late this year, I guess, I haven't been around….
I would have been fine in a T-shirt. That's ok, my vented tech fabric is nice and sweat is good for you…
A rain cloud is following me but from the right angle…I'm on the cool side, the lee of the negligible breeze…I could right a parody of that Cat Stevens song "Moonshadow" called "Rainshadow…"
(I do, in fact, write a parody)
Wow. I have this whole mountain to myself! Just wow. I bet that's how that kid who died last night felt…
I should email my boss…
I should look over my investment options while I have money…
Do I take that apartment or continue to stay with family when I'm here for free…space or money…peace or convenience…
Am I doing what's best for my child…am I doing what's best for me….how mutually exclusive are those things?
Maybe I should just get an RV…or wait till after the holidays…
Maybe I should quit ignoring my slightly injured leg…maybe the pain will go away if I keep ignoring it…
I was supposed to call multiple doctors today and research new insurance plans.

I can do that when I'm-

Suddenly I'm 3 miles up the mountain, sort of accidentally, and realize the next 3 are all downhill, and that my 5 miles turned into a 10K and I don't care what Strava says, there is no way this is not my best 10K ever. And up (and down) a mountain at that. I hate hills. I loathe hills on the road but I suddenly realize my love of mountains overpowers this loathing by far. I suddenly realize I want to run on mountains all the time.

When I check Strava later I have 7 accomplishments including my best 5 mile ever and I could have opened my stride and drastically improved my split time on the downhill stretch but who cares? That was my reward. I pushed myself up and enjoyed the ride down, and still did great, still a few personal records only worth mentioning to other avid runners. And, it's the longest I've run since my half marathon almost 3 months ago right before my "injury." It's only 6 miles, but it's good to be back.

I sit in my car after my cool down, waiting for the endorphin rush to subside a little because it actually makes me feel like I'm in no shape to drive. Is this that lactic acid crash I hear so much about? I think you're supposed to do something about that, but I never do. It feels awesome. It's like what I imagine a morphine drip with a hint of psychedelic mushrooms might be. I wonder why anyone ever does drugs. This is so much better.

Suddenly it's 3:50 and by the time I get anywhere it will be too late to do anything on my list. Maybe an email, maybe a phone call. I was supposed to meet someone, sort of, at some point...

Instead I get coffee and sit down to write. And then it starts pouring outside. I have hated driving in the rain ever since that first accident I had at 16. I still never trust tires and brakes on wet pavement, especially with leaves. Those conditions are meant for pedestrian traffic. Languid walks in the rain alone or with an adventurous loved one, or emotionally driven, angsty, cathartic, empowering bursts of athleticism. So I grab an everything bagel with egg and cheese and head home.

I have so many things to do. So many things. I just spent 5 months far, far away. 6 days a week, 11 hours a day at work; an endless repeat of days in which I attempt to accomplish the same set of tasks over and over till I finally, one day, manage to get them all done and done right. I have been living the movie "Groundhog Day."

I have people to see. So much time to spend with people I've left, and the few I ever really miss. I have a matter of days to coldly pencil them all in. But I need time with me. I have missed me most of all.

I need silence I haven't had in months. I need a whole mountain to myself. So what do I do today? Nothing. Nothing at all, except for 6.2 miles.

My name is Maggie, I'm from Chattanooga, TN, and I'm an archaeologist. I travel about 9 months out of the year for work. I started running in November 2013 because I wanted to be able to get a good workout wherever I am, despite money or access to a hotel gym. My work is physically strenuous but the schedule is unreliable, and I was determined to stay in shape between projects. I couldn't run 100 yards at when I started running, but I soon fell in love. I have now completed 2 half marathons, and have a strenuous 15 mile trail race planned this weekend. My goal to run ultras and beyond, and particularly love tackling mountains.

Remaining Upright
by Michelle Roberts
"What's the matter, honey?"

By the time my father asked me I never even knew the answer. He said when I was a teenager he used to watch as I took on more and more – bigger challenges, harder classes and more after-school activities. He waited on the sidelines for me to meet my match and finally hit a wall I couldn't climb over. He wanted to be there for me when it happened. But he said I never did. I made it over every one.

It was the emotional toll and the stress I put myself under that only he recognized. The fatigue that came from going too long without rest and the tears from putting myself last on the list. He worked overnight shifts as a communications technician at the Space Center and did computer programming on the side to pay for my braces. He knew first-hand about fatigue. Each time he took me aside and forced me to sit still long enough to ask me that question I was a puddle – every time. I'd shake my head and cry after weeks of answering, "I'm fine." Upset over a jumble of so many teen-aged injustices and hurt feelings that I couldn't begin to unravel them. A long talk, some fatherly advice and a few hugs served as my psychological reset. It put me firmly on my feet until the next time I felt overwhelmed.

Two years ago it was my Dad who warned me against attempting my first full marathon.

"People train for those, you know? They don't just show up for a marathon."

Sure I'd finished a few half marathons but a full looked to him like one of those walls he always worried about. Except I knew that in the twenty-five years since high school I'd hit a few all on my own. I'd fallen flat, recovered and survived many times by then. I never saw the walls when I was younger but, in my forties, I knew they were there and they didn't scare me.

I don't remember if I told him I only made it halfway through my first attempt at a marathon in February 2014. I didn't have to say anything. He was always the person I hurried to tell and he knew he'd have seen the medal if I'd earned it. No matter how old I was there would always exist in me the little girl showing off her report card. Only 13.1 miles that day due to an injury but my Moon Jogger friends rallied around me almost immediately and I registered for my next marathon – 26.2 with Donna in Jacksonville February 2015 to financially support women going through breast cancer treatment. With over 1,500 Moon Jogger miles in 2014 I'd worked up to my 20 mile training run/walk in early January and felt ready for my first marathon finish. Sheila Dawe from BC, Canada, was flying in to run with me and my faithful cheerleader, Carolyn Guhman, from New Orleans was bringing her trusty purple pom poms.

Then on January 16th I got the call that my father had suffered a sudden cardiac arrest and was on life support. It was late on a Friday night and he was going to be removed from the machines the next morning. The wind was knocked out of me.

I went through the next couple weeks on autopilot – forcing myself to eat and doing my best to sleep. When it was time for my 24 mile training run I knew I didn't have the strength to remain upright. Thankfully over the years I'd internalized the question my Father used to ask me to check in on my own emotional well-being. I made sure that, mixed with all the ways I thought I needed to contribute to those around me, there was plenty of joy in my life.

Hours spent doing what I loved with the people I loved. I knew what it felt like to run on empty and what it took to fill up my reserves. I'd even learned to rest. To take the time I needed for myself no matter who needed me. If there was ever a time to quiet the goal-driven perfectionist in me this was it. I decided twenty miles would have to do and I'd adjust my training to include

10 miles/6 miles in the weeks ahead.

So many things fell into place in the next few weeks I could feel my father's hands in all of it. My last two longer runs were strong and the heaviness in my heart began to lift. Carolyn told me that if her new granddaughter was born by Monday then she would make the drive to Tallahassee to join me in Jacksonville. Quinn was born Monday night after 9pm and right on time! We drove over Saturday morning to meet Sheila for the Expo with a quick detour in St. Augustine to show off the Nation's Oldest City to our Canadian friend.

Even the weather forecast cooperated by inching up one degree at a time until race day was the perfect high of 55 – sunny with an ocean breeze
The morning of the marathon I had just the right amount of ignorance about everything. I'm usually anxious about doing something for the first time but felt the support of so many friends and an inexplicable confidence about finishing. With Sheila by my side we did intervals along the beachfront road to the cheers of the local community and many grateful breast cancer survivors.

After several miles the course turned onto the beach with the full force of those ocean breezes, 15 mph winds, in our faces and the hard sand under our feet. But what a view! The half marathoners turned back and we wound through shady subdivisions past mile marker 16. By then I was spent and had given up on intervals. We walked as fast as I could manage while keeping tabs on our pace with a silent goal of finishing within the 7 hour window.

At mile 20 we were heading back along the beachfront road. This was my longest distance! I knew after finishing twenty there was no way I wouldn't get those last 6.2 miles. Today was the day I was going to finish my first full marathon – almost exactly one month after losing my father. I thought about how I'd never have the chance to show him my medal and that's when the tears came silently as I put one foot in front of the other.

After passing mile marker 22 I told Sheila, "I can do anything for 4 miles!" She grinned knowing those four are a whole lot different after the previous twenty-two. And after twenty-three miles of gorgeous scenery, palm-lined roads and oak canopies, we turned onto A1A with views of fast food restaurants and gas stations. I realized we were heading toward an onramp.

Um. What?

That's where the ignorance came into play. Begrudgingly I made it up the onramp and onto the highway leading to the finish line at the Mayo Clinic. When I spotted the bridge ahead I asked another runner, "We're not going over that, are we?"

"Mile 25 is at the top and mile 26 is at the bottom. There's no way around it" she explained.

I turned to Sheila knowing it was probably a good thing I didn't pay attention to the course map the night before. She doesn't have much of a taste for profanity.

"You're fu@*&ng kidding me?!" I said, under my breath, and Sheila pretended she didn't hear me. But I knew my Navy father would've found it completely appropriate given the circumstances.

Sheila waited a few minutes before adding, "I'm going to say this now because you might not want to hear it later. I'm really proud of you! You did amazing!" "Thanks," as I stared straight ahead but managed a smile, "and please don't talk to me while we're on the bridge." Actually, I'm not sure I said please.

But the bridge was almost worth it when we reached the top. To know that mile 26 was in our sights and the glorious downhill was ahead.

"Ok, we have time for a couple more stories." I told Sheila who'd been generously entertaining me with tales of Ultras and Canada and coulees for hours already.

As we rounded the off-ramp and were heading into the finish line I saw those wonderful purple pom poms and Carolyn's big New Orleans smile cheering us on. Our Moon Jogger friend, Robyn Hershberger, had volunteered at the finish since 7am just so she could put the ribbons around our necks. And she did. And we all smiled. Until Carolyn caught me crying and we hugged. She understood.

I did it! In 6 hours and 57 minutes.

As confident as I felt that morning and with everything that happened in the month before, this was one wall I wasn't quite sure I could climb. Until I actually did.

ABOUT: Michelle Roberts lives in Tallahassee, Florida, with her husband, Paul, and two children, Ashleigh (12) and Philip (9). She ran her first 5k in October of 2012, her first half marathon in February of 2013 and her first full marathon in February 2015. She was diagnosed with Bipolar Disorder in 2001 and maintains a healthy balance without the use of medication thanks to a job she loves, a supportive family, regular exercise, her writing and therapy. A wonderful life of "Both Hills and Valleys".

"The marvelous richness of human experience would lose something of rewarding joy if there were no limitations to overcome. The hilltop hour would not be half so wonderful if there were no dark valleys to traverse." Helen Keller

LIVING WITH LYMPHOEDEMA
by Lynne Harness

In the United Kingdom, March 2nd-6th is lymphoedema awareness week. This prompted me to share my own story of living with lymphoedema. Lymphoedema is a visible swelling that develops because there is a problem with the lymph drainage system. The lymph system is no longer able to drain away all the fluid and waste products that have built up in the tissues. The swelling that develops when the lymph system cannot work properly is not just made up of fluid, but also contains material such as fat cells. In time the skin can lose its soft feeling and become hard due to fibrous changes, or rubbery because of the build up of fat cells. The swelling is usually in an arm or leg but can affect more than one part of the body.

I was diagnosed with breast cancer in 2006. Lymph nodes were removed during surgery and I also received radiotherapy. Both treatments can cause lymphoedema, which I developed soon after.

I visit the specialist lymphoedema nurse annually now for review and measurements, and I am pleased to report that at present I appear to be managing my condition effectively.

I find that the slightest weight gain can impact on my lymphoedema and I need to keep my weight down. My running and walking helps with this. I also choose loose sleeved clothing that is comfortable and not constrictive.

Every 4 weeks a physiotherapy aid who has had specialist training in the technique visits me at home and I have manual lymphatic drainage. This is a massage which moves the lymph out of the swollen areas into parts of the body where it can channel away normally.

I wear a compression sleeve and glove on my left arm and hand, this applies pressure to the skin and provides support to reduce swelling. These compression garments improve the effect of exercise by helping the muscles massage fluid out through the existing lymphatic vessels.

Cellulitis is an infection caused by bacteria that affects the skin and the tissues beneath it. The immune system in the swollen part of the body is not working as well, and cannot fight the infection. Cellulitis is often one of the main reasons why lymphoedema develops or gets worse, and so good skin care is important. This includes daily moisturising, not getting sunburn, protecting the skin from thorns and scratches when gardening, and cleaning and treating any stings, bites, burns or cuts promptly.

My lymphoedema is also affected by long haul air journeys and I need to wear my compression garments, and elevate my arm when travelling.

If any other Moon Joggers are affected by lymphoedema, I would be pleased to hear from you.

My name is Lynne Harness and I am 54 years of age. I live in the beautiful county of Yorkshire in England. I am a granny-nanny to my four grand-children and provide childcare when their parents work. I grew up in a family where there was always a pet dog so I have always enjoyed walking and the outdoors. I have been running regularly since I was in my 20s

Every Step Counts
by Catherine Campbell

I think of this especially on long runs when I am doing 10/30 run/walk/run intervals and I begin to get a little tired. It takes about 26 steps for the 10 second interval. That doesn't seem like much but as I silently count down the steps I feel more in control. When I first started running, six years ago, and was first being coached by my daughter, Sheila, she told me, "Think of control and comfort". While comfort is a relative thing, control is necessary and achievable, I think. "Control" is of both a physical and mental effort. Part of the control is having a routine, motivation and drive to be committed to continue with a training program, even when you don't feel like it or excuses are plentiful.

I'm in no position to give advice except when running with my friend, who is four years younger than me and still a beginner runner. She isn't a regular runner, but would like to be, but she has health issues to deal with. Most of us have health issues of some sort. I have a disease, Sarcoidosis, that I "work around". Last year I broke my fibula in 2 places and was in an air cast for 9 weeks. After 1 week of immobilization, I went for walks anyway…cast and all. I didn't walk far, but I walked every day. I knew how quickly muscle strength diminishes at my age so I "worked around" being in a cast. Acquaintances at my seniors' club think I'm foolish to be running at all. But my doctors are proud of me and encourage me to keep running. So, why not? I don't go fast and I don't go far, but I go!

Right now I'm training for my first half marathon on May 3rd, 2015. My training for this event last year was interrupted by slipping on wet wood stairs and breaking my leg. It had nothing to do with running despite what all my fellow seniors thought. This year I am getting e-coaching with Jeff Galloway, which is great, just as is the "home" coaching with Sheila. I like running with Coach Sheila because I don't have to think about pace or distance or water breaks or "Gu" time. She tells me "slow it down a bit", "next walk break take a drink ", and when to re-fuel.

I started running 6 years ago when I was 72 years old. Before that I had done a lot of long distance walking events. In England 315 kilometers on The Wainwright's Trail from St. Bees Head to Robin Hood's Bay, coast to coast. I also ventured to Holland for the Four Days March from Nijmegen, where I walked 30 km a day for a total of 120 kms in 4 days. My final European walking adventure was the el Camino de Santiago in Spain where I walked 150 km. I have also participated in 10 long distance walking events from 50 to 60 kilometers in a single day, here in BC. Canada. All this walking history but never running. Runners didn't look as if they were having much fun. I didn't know about endorphins.

Cheering for Sheila at marathon finish lines made me wonder how hard could it be? Maybe someone would cheer for me at the finish line! As it turned out my children cheered...except when they were running the same race and determined not to let their mother beat them. Children and grandchildren all beat me time-wise but I'm the only member of my family that won gold in my age category. Not that I bragged about it....oh no. Two more years and I will be in the 80-84 age category. Look out world, here I come! Meanwhile, back at being humble, I carry on doing what I can to stay fit and hope that my few steps count and help Moon Joggers reach our goal.

Bio: Catherine Campbell has 3 children and 4 grandchildren. She is retired and living next door to her daughter/coach Sheila in beautiful Nanaimo, B.C. Canada. Catherine is 78 years young and looking forward to running, at least until the next age category. Since learning to run in 2008, she has run in four 5 kms., six 8 kms, and four 10 kms. Her crowning glory was in one of her early races where she won her age category in the B.C. Championship 5 km Road Race and received a beautiful trophy and cash reward.

Run Fit With A Friend (Mate)
By Coach Richard Rykbos

Hello fellow Moon Joggers, as some of you know I am Coach Rykbos and my lovely wife Ilene. We began this journey to rack up mileage to the outer ends of the universe back in September when Perry ran across the U.S.A.
While I am a fitness enthusiast and Certified Personal trainer among other titles, there is one thing that is for sure. I believe in the TEAM Spirit when it comes to getting your best results in any physical exercise program, so I wanted to focus on the Team and doing this journey with a friend.
One of my favorite books says two are better than one and a three strand cord is stronger... With over a decade in the wellness industry and coming from a 300 pound fat, sick and dying position I can only tell you that movement works. When done with an accountability partner or friend to keep the motivation high it tends to have a better success rate.

Like a marathon or ultra marathon having the support of a friend really creates a sense of I can do this and keeps you going. Running with a determination and commitment that NO One is Left behind is a great way to help another win. Take our Tough Mudders where the condition of the run or climate are up in the air, and while you train for it and do all you can to be prepared, the unknown can take a team member out. That is when sticking it out together and encouraging others to keep putting one foot in front of the other helps to finish strong no matter what comes, because you had another to lift your spirits and believe in you. SO many times we have seen people go on to even better wellness goals and set records and personal best for themselves and encourage others.

Take Jeannie here to the left who began with us and Fit Friends at 320 Pounds. With six kids it is not easy to balance life family and regain health and wellness. But from a first start of a walk/jog and the encouragement of friends she has lost over 150 pounds and now coaches others to live a well life using walking and running as a way to get healthy.

Partnering with a Audacious Dream and becoming motivated and develop lifelong friendships with running. Ilene began her journey in running with a few steps (Her 1st Mile) with a little Kiwi making his way across the USA. What started out as supporting her husband and his ambitions became a believable I Can Do It Attitude of running. Because of this new friend and his encouragement and determination she began running 1 mile a day while he was out there and by the time he had finished she was up to 4 miles a day. Yes a friend can change the direction of your life for the healthier.

Lifting and encouraging you through a recovery from injury or setbacks. Having an accountability partner or like-minded friend can keep giving you the slightest praise and accolades when you just have lost your motivation. Seeing their likes on social media, and email or private message can really encourage them to take that initial step and get back in the game. This last December 2014 I had exactly that, an injury from some of the extreme training I do and then an added cough that caused me to dislodge a rib that was not discovered for 6 weeks... So I went from running 75 to 100 miles a week to barely moving, it was then this true warrior and friend continued to encourage me to Keep it up Mate! Doing good even when I was only doing a mile or less.

So in closing of this blog for our journey to the ends of the worlds and beyond, let me just encourage you to always be aware of those you are running with, and if they need a hand be ready to give it... It can make the difference in whether this person continues or falls so far behind they feel they cannot start again. We All Need a Running Friend and that is why the Moon Joggers is so much a Family... Even recently Ilene and I had not posted for a while and a Fellow Moon Jogger gave a shout out looking for us! That is what we do for each other... Keep setting Audacious Goals and Have Fun on Your Journey with Friends.

Strength and Honor
Coach Rykbos

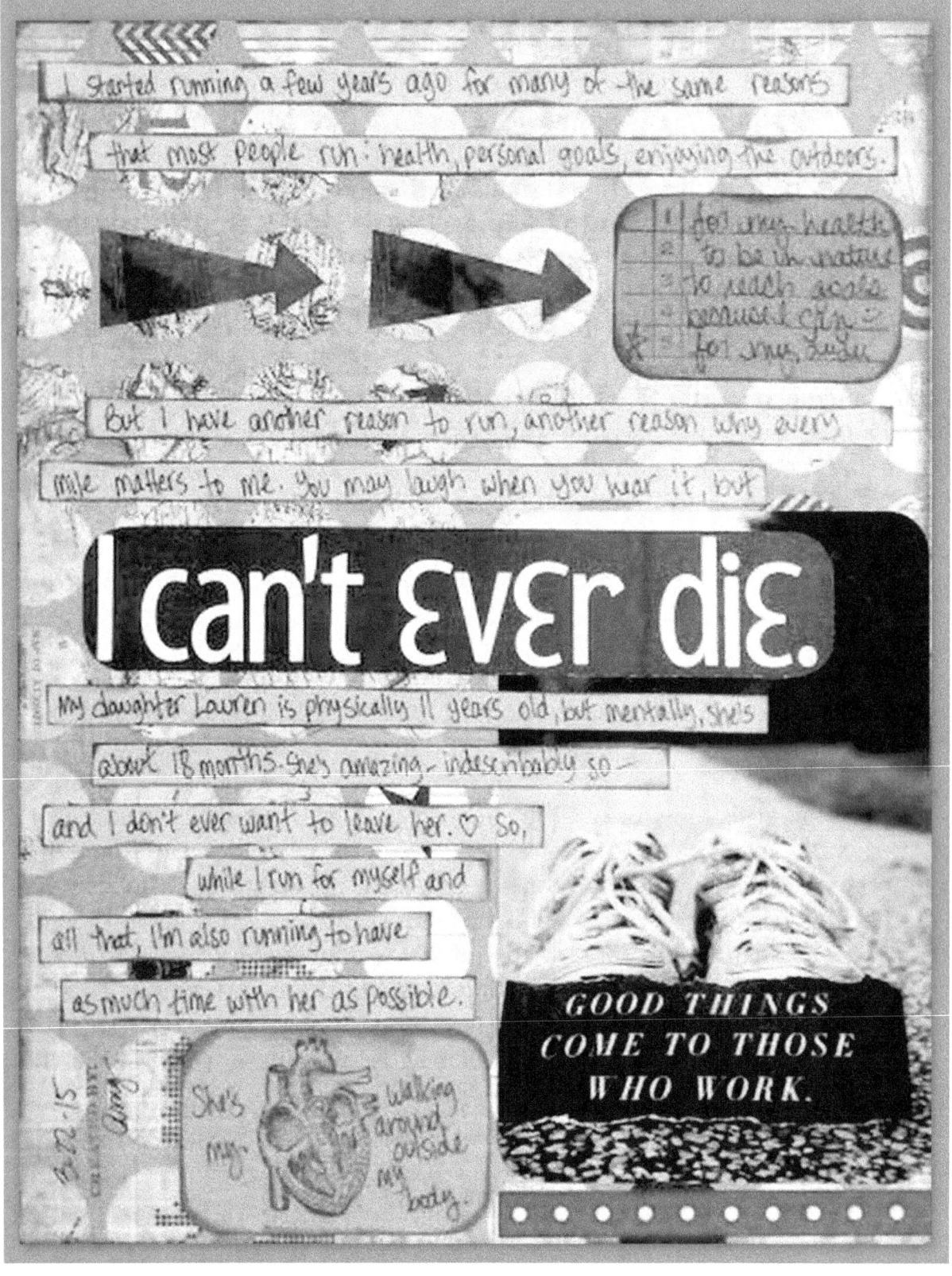

I started running a few years ago for many of the same reasons that most people run: health, personal goals, enjoying the outdoors.

1. for my health
2. to be in nature
3. to reach goals
4. because I can
5. for Mrs. Taylor

But I have another reason to run, another reason why every mile matters to me. You may laugh when you hear it, but

I can't ever die.

My daughter Lauren is physically 11 years old, but mentally, she's about 18 months. She's amazing, indescribably so –

and I don't ever want to leave her. ♡ So, while I run for myself and all that, I'm also running to have as much time with her as possible.

She's my heart walking around outside my body.

GOOD THINGS COME TO THOSE WHO WORK.

My Reason to Run
Collage by Amy Preneta

I recently turned 40 and have been running for three years. I live in and love Cleveland, Ohio. I used to work for the federal government, but gave it up to raise my triplet daughters who decided to join us at 24 weeks instead of holding out 'till 40. I've run lots of 5Ks, 10Ks, and halfs, but I think 10K is my preferred distance. I run in my neighborhood and in our wonderful county park system. I've worked through a lot of problems and feelings while out on the trails. In December, I got a new running partner, a sweet pointer named Mali. She's faster than me!

In case you can't read the writing in the picture above, it read:
 I started running a few years ago for many of the same reasons that most people run: health, personal goals, enjoying the outdoors.
1. For my health
2. To be in nature
3. To reach goals
4. Because I can
*5. For my LuLu

But I have another reason to run, another reason why every mile matters to me. You may laugh when you hear it, but I can't ever die. My daughter Lauren is physically 11 years old, but mentally, she's about 18 months. She's amazing – indescribably so – and I don't ever want to leave her. So, while I run for myself and all that, I'm also running to have as much time with her as possible. She's my heart walking around outside my body.

Every Mile Matters
– Tina Bond

I have come to a difficult decision. I think I am going to give up running. The thrill is gone. Pretty, big, shiny medals have lost their lure. Training has become a chore. I don't enjoy eating all the food. I especially don't like that my pants don't fit me anymore! If you believe that…. APRIL FOOLS!!!!!

The thrill isn't gone. I had the biggest thrill when I FINALLY reached a huge goal of mine in January. Since I started long distance running I've wanted to run a 2:45 half. I ran the Celebration Half this year, in perfect running conditions, without the use of intervals and no walk breaks of any kind, and finished the race in 2:32:24!!! I was elated and on a runners high for at least a week! I started long distance running in 2012 (running in general in 2007), so it took me about 2 years to finally hit my goal. I blew that goal out of the water!!

As far as medals, I love medals. Normally I do not sign up for 5 or 10k races because they typically don't give out race bling, but I'm seeing more and more races doing just that! And some of the bling is really pretty! If I can find a 5 or 10k that is reasonably priced that also gives out medals (that's not too far of a drive), I'm more likely to sign up. I love looking at my medals and the memories they bring back for each of my races. That's why I love race medals.

Training can be challenging at times! We all have our moments, but right now for me training is fun. Sure there are days that I don't want to get out there, but I usually feel better after a run. I've had weeks where I didn't get out there as much as I wanted or should have and I look back on those weeks with regret. If I had just gone out and done 2 miles! If you do nothing but go out and walk 2 miles a day, 5 days a week, that's 10 miles a week, 40 miles a month, 480 miles a year!! Sometimes I'll go out for a 3 mile run in the morning and a 2 mile walk in the afternoon. That ends up being a 5 mile day!

It's so important to understand how, in our Moon Jogger group, every mile does matter!!

If you know me, you know that one of the reasons why I run is so I can eat all the food!! You knew from the moment of reading that sentence this had to be some kind of joke! I love being able to go out for a long run and not feel guilty for wanting to eat ice cream or indulge with cupcakes, or have an ice cream cupcake! I do not go overboard because there are still limits to what I can and should eat. Running allows me to be able to indulge in the things I love to eat. So there's no way I can stop running.

As far as my pants not fitting... well that relates more to running than eating (most of the time!!)!! I've come to learn that 'skinny jeans' are not for athletes. My calves are too big for skinny jeans. When I put on a pair of skinny jeans I feel like my calves are about to bust out of them! Even my thighs don't feel quite right in regular jeans. Some women athletes even have problems with their booty not fitting right in jeans. I do not know if men have the same issues. Sorry guys! I should probably ask Jim if he has these issues, but he doesn't wear skinny jeans. Alas, it is good to have a problem with clothes fitting but not because of weight gain, but because I am gaining MUSCLE! I wish I could say the same for button down shirts, but that's another topic for another day.

I guess the moral of this April Fools Tale is to keep moving. Keep moving so you can get miles in. So you can eat all the food. So you don't fit into skinny jeans. And don't forget about getting the shiny bling.

Tina lives in Winter Garden with her husband and fellow Moon Jogger, Jim. When she's not jet setting across the country with her job or running, or training for a race, or recovering from a race, she enjoys reading, photography, movies, music and going to Disney!!

Every Mile Matters
by Carol-Lee Holland

When my BF challenged me to run a 5k with her 3 years ago, I had no idea what it would do to my life. Let me set the stage…I was living in a new city with only my hubby. We were learning about the new city by eating our way through all the new restaurants…hence gaining weight along the way. I had never run, felt I couldn't run, but she wanted me to run a Disney race in February 2013 for a girls weekend, as an excuse to be able to go visit. She gave me almost 10 months to train, and I told her I would try. Luckily, I worked with a bunch of the most supportive people that I have ever met, and many of them are runners. I got advice, support, help, and shoulders to lean on. I signed up for a 5k locally so that I could motivate myself to train, and when I crossed that first finish line, I KNEW I could do it! I called BF and said I would meet her in Disney…she then informed me that we would be running the half marathon, and not the 5k! SHE KNEW I could do it, and that I was hooked! Let the training begin!

Since the day I started training for that 5k, May 1, 2012, I haven't stopped. I've changed my eating habits, lost close to 25#, wake up thinking about my next run, go to sleep thinking of my next run. I have injured myself and healed. I have learned what to eat before a run. I've learned how to hydrate properly. I have learned that "poop" is a typical conversation amongst runners. But mostly, I have accomplished more than I thought was possible. I have now run 17 half marathons, and I'm not done…I continue to push myself. I have dropped over 30 minutes off my first half, but I am still trying to reach my goal of a sub 2:15…I'm hoping 2015 will be my year, but if not, I will keep trying. I have also decided to run my first full this year, and that is scary! Scary because I know it will be hard and require an amount of discipline that I'm not positive I have in me; however, I feel I am really at a point of giving this a shot and making these miles count.

When I joined Moon Joggers in December 2012, I didn't know what to expect. Tina and I talked about it and decided to give it a try…1000 miles in a year? What the heck! Well, I have yet to reach that goal but I'm not giving up. This is where the "Every Mile Counts" attitude comes in. Every mile matters to me because I do not want to go back to that overweight, unhealthy, inactive person. I have watched my mom grow older, and less active, and it hurts me. I do not want to be that way…I have a new grand-baby, and I want to be active when her kids are born…not sitting in a chair because my muscles and bones will not allow me to get on the floor to play, or take them for a walk, or push them on swings. I will continue to push myself each year to reach the 1000 and when I finally reach that goal, I will make a new goal. The goals keep me motivated, the races (& bling) keep me addicted, and the friendships I've made keep me smiling!

My husband, Steve, joined me running about a year into my journey. It is nice having someone close to share the ups and downs of my runs, and he is as addicted as I am. Together we understand what it takes, but we also have our own goals and mind-set. He's much faster, so we never run together, but he is one of my biggest supporters in this journey.

So my journey of a thousand miles began with one step…and each step counts, as does each mile…Keep moving forward people, don't go backwards…nobody's got time for that!

Every Mile Matter
by Barbara Corn

Hi! I've run and been active my whole life but about 7 years ago my bones ached so bad from arthritis that I no longer ran for at least 3 or 4 years. I put on weight and was not happy. I changed my diet to an alkaline diet and no more pain. I was being poisoned by processed foods. I began to run 5 ks again and it was fun. Last year around Easter I almost lost my husband to sepsis. He was in the hospital for a month. I would work, go to the hospital and visit him while he was comatose, and go home with so much frustration that I ran and bicycled til midnight. I decided that life was short and I needed to complete my bucket list. Last year I did 15 events. My first 10k, warrior dash, triathlon sprint among some. This year I'm signed up for triathlons, obstacle runs, 5k's cause they are fun, 10k's, and my first half marathon on May 3rd. I don't want to have regrets later. Thank God my husband is still alive and my life is blessed.

Why Every Mile Matters
By Eric Clifford

Why every mile matters. I could sit here and tell you all some great (ehh) tale about how I needed to get back into shape after an accident. Or, I could tell you about how I'm always about sports and sports is my life! Or even about how I was lost, empty and needed something to fill the hole that was inside me. All of that would be true to an extant but the real reason is that I just didn't have anything better to do. All my friends stopped playing ball (softball, football, basket...) "I've got this with the family." or "I'm doing that with the family." I have the kids blah blah blah... You see, being the first one of my friends to get married and have kids I know all that is all bullshit. There's always time for yourself.

So after a couple years of doing nothing and going from 175/180lbs to 195/200lbs and feeling like my head was going to pop when I bent over to tie my shoes I was like "This sucks. I have got to start doing something." What can you do that's a good exercise and that you can do alone... (light bulb) Running! So I started. Three miles a day in about 40 minutes. I was gassed, sore and couldn't stop thinking about what the hell happened to me. But I stuck with it and pushed myself to where I'm pretty happy with my distance and speed (most of the time).

Running is part of my life now. But sometimes it becomes my life and I'm not overly happy with that. There must be balance. You need to stay happy or at least not dread the idea of running. If you plan on running races it's all that much more important. I run for myself. I run to stay in shape to do things. I run so when I go to the show the seat is reasonably comfortable (well that was before most theaters put in oversized seats) and so I can get on a plane and not be squeezed in the seat. I want to be able to work around the house landscaping, or building new decks or putting up walls... I run because I want a life. I'm selfish that way. I know that as long as I can do what needs to be done and then some, everything else will fall into place. I'll be able to take care of my family, my house, my work doing side jobs (albeit my acting/extra work is pretty easy). I needed something to do so I could do something. Every Mile Matters because they bring me closer to where and what I want to be.

A Day in the Life when Every Mile Matters
By Sheila Dawe

March 26th, 2015

5:00 pm. Arrived in Boise, Idaho. I got picked up at the airport by my good friend Natalie. We are both entered in a new race for the both of us – Pickled Feet Time Runs (48, 24, 12, 6 hour and 100 mile): Natalie in the 100 mile event and me in the 24 hour event.

10:00 pm. Did I take a sleeping pill or not, I remember opening the bottle but I don't remember taking a pill. To err on the side of caution, I decided I must have taken the pill.

March 27th, 2015

12:30 am. Or not.

6:00 am. It is time to get ready despite having plenty of time. Natalie starts at 10:00 am and is already anxious to get going. I don't start until 6 pm…it is going to be a long day despite my very late start.

9:00 am. We arrive at the Eagle Island State Park and find the main pavilion. Natalie picks up her race package and I stare at the 48 hour participants that are presently in their 15th hour. I am a bit shocked by the fact that they already look very tired. What I did not know was that they had suffered a cold foggy night.

10:00 am. All the 100 mile contestants are to start. They have 32 hours to complete 40 laps of the 2.5 mile loop. Go Natalie go – but not too fast, it is predicted to be a warm day. Now I have to focus on staying off my feet, drinking fluids, eating and resting…this will be the strangest race for me.

3:00 pm. Oh the carnage has begun. It is very hot on the course and all the runners are starting to look like they are overheating. I begin to make myself useful by trying to help fill water bottles with ice and water and aid as much as I can. The hours are slowly ticking by, I can't believe I have been here all day.

6:00 pm. Finally we get to line up for our start. I am wearing my "Streak Runner's International" jersey and got the usual comment, "Do you run naked?" I smile and say "No but this will be day 389 and 390". And we are off…yay!!

8:30 pm. After a spectacular sunset and with dusk settling in I finally turn on the head lamp. My goal is to try to continue my run/walk throughout the night. In the past, with most Ultras, I have always defaulted to walking once it has become dark. This time being so fresh, it is a great opportunity to practice my night running.

March 28th, 2015

2:00 am. Sheila is up and boom Sheila is down. Yikes I am falling. Knee hits ground, then left breast, left shoulder and right hand. I see from my head lamp my bottle rolling along the path. I sat and semi hyperventilated due to the shock of hitting the ground. I took inventory: my chest hurt a little and my hand hurt a whole lot. From here on in I would not be able to use my right hand and would carry my water bottle only in the left.

2:20 am. Upon arriving back at the aid station, I sat down and nearly started to cry, as I felt sorry for myself. The race director came up to me and asked if I was okay. I told her of the fall but said I thought I was fine and asked for a coffee. The black elixir was very comforting and just the boost I needed to get my butt off of the chair and back out into the dark.

3:30 am. A volunteer asked me if I would like company. I told her I was only walking but trying to walk fast, she said that would be fine. She entertained me with stories of how she is doing seven 100 mile events this year with the Grand Circle Trail Series. We talked of so many different things during this lap, I felt like a made a true friend (although I still can't remember her name) and it was just the boost I needed to power me on for the rest of this journey.

7:00 am. As I came into the aid station, the wind suddenly picked up to hurricane force gusts, tents, tables and signs were flying. I went into the main tent to get extra layers as I was feeling chilled. The ground looked very inviting but as the wind whipped around my ankles, I knew the best plan of action was to keep on moving.

9:00 am. Natalie and I had constantly seen each other throughout this race. I knew she would be walking at this stage and ironically we both had the same idea to wait for each other and join forces. As we walked her final three laps together, and the morning began to heat up, it was so nice to change my focus from "me" to "her" and getting her to the finish.

12:46 pm. Natalie finishes her 100 mile in 2nd place female, 5th overall in 26:46 – I was very proud of her and glad I could share a small part of it. I am at mile 60, my primary goal is to get three more laps done to complete the distance I was supposed to do for my ultra-training.

2:00 pm. I tried to run again for a short stretch but for fear of burning myself out, I opted to keep to a fast walk, especially since I was passing some of the 48 hour runners. As I walked, I caught up to some other competitors and I mused out loud, "I wish I knew what place I was in". A fellow competitor checked his I-phone and told me I am tied for 3rd female with two competitors close behind. "Thanks, and see ya". I said as I picked up my pace – talk about your boost of energy.

3:30 pm. Natalie has returned, it was so good to see a friendly face. I told her the scenario. She checked the standings and told me...you need 2 more laps to secure your place.

4:30 pm. I lie down in the main tent. There is excruciating pain in my ribs when I lie down, so I get up and do that one more insurance lap.

5:15 pm. There is a short course (.28 mile) for the final hour. Natalie convinces me to give it a go for a lap. It was so enjoyable, I did 3 more laps before the magic hour of 6 pm finally arrived.

Post-script. Upon arrival back home, I went to see the doctor. Nothing was broken in the hand although it remained swollen and painful for over 3 weeks. I had a hairline fracture in one rib, but I did not affect my running only my resting. Must keep on keeping on.

Biography: Sheila is 50 years old, living in Nanaimo, B.C. Being single without any kids leads to an active life filled with lots of running and travelling. She is currently training for two big events in 2015: Squamish 50/50 (50 miles on Aug. 22nd and 50 km on Aug. 23rd) and Lost Souls Ultra 100 mile (Sept. 11th and 12th). Both these event she attempted and DNFed in 2014. This year she has a different training program and is determined to do her best, have fun and hopefully complete these events.

Every Mile Matters, Especially at the Boston Marathon
By Shirlee Webb

Boston Marathon has proven two times now that things can change in a twinkling of an eye. Both times I have run it the weather was forecast a week out to be the perfect weather for a marathon and then within a couple of days before the race, has changed from one extreme of heat three years ago and to the extreme of cold, wet, and windy as warned in an email the day before the race this year.

What I have learned from both of these experiences is that the one thing you can always count on in life is CHANGE! The most important principle I learned is to be unchanged by change. It is what it is -so be it- I realized I needed to keep the same desires and goals I had made for under the best of circumstances, yet be willing to not have the same outcome I had hoped for if circumstances changed. I no longer had the ideal I had hoped for. I realized we can set ourselves up for disappointment and failure if one can't rise to the "changed occasion."

I knew before I ran this marathon that I had decided it would be my last, I have felt a need to quit while I am ahead. I love half marathons and hope to run them til I am called Home, but I also know that these long runs will sooner or later have an effect on me for the worse and in some ways, this run did. I had a cancer scare the first two months of this year and I wasn't able to do anything and I felt that lack of training in this race.

Two weeks later I continue to feel extremely tired and I have gotten some of the physical challenges back that I experienced with the cancer scare. So I know this is the correct decision for me to make. As life winds down in later years I am sure I will make decisions required in rethinking running even half's although I hope not too soon.

Boston Marathon is always exhilarating because of the great people we are surrounded by throughout the whole race. Those great folks who volunteer by the thousands and the great support we receive all along the way by the public. I didn't even listen to my music this time because of the enthusiastic noise all along the route from Hopkinton to Boston. It never let down–they were getting as wet as us and the wind and cold was there for them too.

I experienced the great human spirit of endurance as I passed the fellow with Muscular Dystrophy who took 20 hours to run and was that long in the pouring rain. I was also very humbled by the two blind fellows who had guides and were joyfully running alongside of me several times. I sometimes heard the words in my mind "God forgive me when I whine."

Like three years ago it proved to be a run of endurance. Last time 93 degree heat from the get go and this time, the very cold, wet, and windy weather. I had to change my four hour or less goal and I had to decide just to do my best and just finish. Even though circumstances changed, I felt complete joy when I finished no matter how ugly it was!

I am grateful and thankful to again learn the lesson that you can always do what you set out to do by not changing yourself nor the desires of your heart and finish anything you desire to do even if the circumstances change. When things become hard, don't become hard with them. Find the joy in the journey whatever it gives you. I feel gratitude alone that I can still run at my age and find such great joy in it.

About Shirlee: She ran her first marathon when she was 45 years old, after giving birth to eight children. She is now a 63 year old grandmother of 13 grandchildren, plus one on the way. She has battled depression and raised a severely mentally ill son. When she first started running she barely made it around the block before she stopped, but she kept getting up each morning and gaining distance a little at a time. When she was 60 she ran the Boston marathon for the first time, in the hottest weather on record, 90+ degrees. Today, at age 63 and 1/2, she ran Boston in the coldest weather, 43 degrees, and finished in 5 hours. She said that today it rained the entire time she ran and it was just as hard as running in the heat. If anyone ever tells you that you can't do it, just remember this, YOU CAN. When the voice in your head tells you to give up and quit, you tell that voice, NO WAY! We were born to do hard things. YOU CAN DO HARD THINGS!

Every Mile Matters
Amber Hadigan

May 11, 2013. I laced up my running shoes for the first time. I was 204 pounds and wore a size 18 pants. I downloaded a couch to 5K app, as I had signed up for a 5K race exactly eight weeks later as motivation. That day, I could hardly run to the end of my driveway.

—

I heard the call up the stairs once again. It was about 11pm, and I had to get up at 5am for school the next day, so I was already in bed. Yet, for some reason, my mom felt the need to yell from her chair, up the stairs, for either me or my brother to wake up, come downstairs, and change the TV channel for her. She was too lazy to get up and do it herself.

My entire high school career was like this. My mom wanted someone to serve her and do all her chores for her, while she sat on her recliner. It was always a frustrating situation for both my brother and me. I got up early for school and he had to be to work at 5am.

I think, by the time I was in high school, my mom just gave up. She worked a job she absolutely hated, but really needed because it paid enough for her to support herself and us. She worked all day, and when she came home, she had nothing left to give. She was overweight and chose to not do anything about it. There was a not-so-secret stash of candy and chips by her chair that we weren't supposed to touch.

I watched my mom eat and sit for years. Her knees started to go and she couldn't even walk the stairs of our townhome to take a shower every day. Yet, for some reason, she never did anything about being fat. I think she actually took pride in it. She used the word fat and talked about being fat like it made her special. Back in those days, it was very rare to see an overweight person.

I loved my mother, but I always knew that there was something slightly wrong with the way she conducted her life. It wasn't a conscious awareness, but a nagging feeling in the back of my mind, one that would pop up just before sleep, when the thoughts about the meaning of life hit this adolescent. I couldn't articulate it at the time, but as I grew into adulthood, I began to understand.

I swore that I would not be like my mother. There was something sad and just a little bit desperate about the way she lived her life. When I was in my 20s, I talked about not wanting to be her. Even when it was hard, I worked on completing goals I had set for myself, such as going to college and getting an advanced degree. I explored activities and was rarely home.

—

Fast forward about fifteen years, to May 11th. What spurred my decision to lace up my shoes, pull out my iPod, and trudge down the road, even though I could barely catch my breath?

My worst fear had come true. I had turned into my mother. I was spiraling out of control, straight into a pit of depression and desperation. At over 200 pounds, I felt uncomfortable in my body. I worked a job I absolutely hated. After working all day, I came home defeated, too tired to even get up off the couch. I developed a terrible sugar addiction. I looked in the mirror and saw the woman I had become, and I hated her.

I toyed with the idea of running for years. I was a track kid in school, but hadn't really run for over twenty years. But something changed when I looked in the mirror. 39 years old, overweight, and couldn't fit into my own clothes. It was time to stop the cycle.

Reading the paper, I saw an ad for an inaugural 5K race during the July 4th weekend. On a whim, I signed up. Now I had money invested, so I had to follow through. I downloaded a couch to 5K app, and on May 11, I went out for the first time.

I thought I would die. My body was not used to moving, let alone running. But I refused to give up. Up at 5am, I would go out and complete my run/walk intervals faithfully, three times a week for the next eight weeks.
An amazing thing happened. I started to be able to run a little longer. When I couldn't run for a minute the first day I went out, by week 6 I could go twenty minutes without stopping! Although I couldn't complete a full 3.1 miles yet, I felt I had accomplished something.

On race day, I thought I would die. It was about 100 degrees and the course was sunny, but I didn't give up. I learned about the supportive nature of the running community. Two women talked to me before the race, cheering me on. My husband came down to watch me cross the finish line. And though I walked some of the course, the feeling of crossing the finish line was something incredible. I wanted to feel it again.

I was hooked. Although training was hard, racing was my savior. I ran 4 5Ks that first year. Then I trained for a half marathon, then a marathon. And although I suffered an injury that sidelined me for 9 weeks, I never gave up faith that running was changing my life.

I could see it in the mirror. I was happier. My clothes fit better. The scale crept down into the ones. And, for the first time in many years, I had a motivation to improve my life. Since I started running, I also started working toward other goals I had dreamed about. I quit the job I hated and became a freelance writer. I began taking creativity coaching classes and want to teach adult education. Each day, I make steps toward the life I want to live. I believe that running spurred all these changes in my life.

Every mile I run proves that I can work hard.
Every mile I run proves that I can set a goal and achieve it.
Every mile I run proves that I am stronger than I was yesterday.
Every mile I run strengthens my perseverance muscle.
Every mile run proves that I am alive!

I don't really know what happened to my mother. She gave up on life when she was about my age. She still may be living, but she does not participate in life.

 As for me, I started living at age 39, when I started running. My 40s will be my best years yet!

Amber Hadigan currently lives in Hyde Park, NY with her husband John and her two cats, Sobe and Scrappy. Originally from Wisconsin, she has lived in many different states. Now settled, she spends her time working, freelance writing, and writing and performing folk music. A runner as a child, she began running again in May 2013 and has rediscovered the peace and joy running gives her.

A Month Ago I Became A Marathon...2 Years Later
By Tara Chavanne

"But guess what....a month ago I became a marathoner (a Big Sur Marathoner)....and I am planning on going back in 2015 to kick Big Sur's butt!! I got this."

Those were the last words I wrote about the Big Sur Marathon 2013. It is now 2 years later and I AM a Big Sur Marathoner 2 times over. But the big question is, did I kick Big Sur's butt or did Big Sur kick mine?!?!

To start with, I came up with a few goals going into this second race. #1 No Tears (you would think this would be easy to accomplish, but if you read the first recap...it's not). #2 Big Sur PR (faster than 4:58:18). #3 Marathon PR (faster than Space Coast 4:35:37). #4 All time PR goal of 4:30:00 and, the most important goal #5 HAVE FUN!

In order for me to obtain my most important goal, I convinced (suckered) fellow Moon Jogger Rebecca DeVall to run her very first marathon with me. There ended up being four Moon Joggers running Big Sur, Carolyn Guhman ran the 21 miler, Dallas Millican ran the 10.6 miler and we had a guest appearance from our Fearless Leader, Angie, cheering us on at the finish line.

Even though Rebecca and I live on opposite coasts, we had a great 9 months of training together, stressing together, and getting excited together to run one of the hardest marathons in the country. We both had minor running issues;

Rebecca's hip had been hurting during long runs and my hamstring was still not 100% since I injured it during my first Big Sur adventure. We decided to run the race together (with the caveat that if one of us was having the race of our life....or wanted to die....the other could run their own race). I knew having a running partner with equal running abilities (and sarcastic nature) would be what would carry me to that finish line with a smile on my face (Tara 1, Big Sur 0).

A week before the race, like normal, crazed runners, the Moon Jogger contingent started discussing the weather and how it was supposed to be cold (for California), rainy (unlike California) with wind speeds of 14 mph (just blah, California)...not the best running weather. As it turned out, we had PERFECT temperatures. The race started in the upper 40s and by the time we crossed the finish line it was in the 70s. BEAUTIFUL! The wind...well...that was another story. Although I didn't think it was THAT bad, (compared to how I thought it was the last time), afterwards we found out that the winds were some of the worst in the races history (Tara 1, Big Sur 1). All I have to say is Rebecca, Carolyn and I are Rock Stars for killing those winds going up to Hurricane Point (Tara 2, Big Sur 1)!

Let me back track a bit.....on the Friday we arrived in Monterey, we took a road trip to Big Sur. I wanted to see the course again. As we drove up, I had two completely opposite reactions. First, was the reminiscing...mostly...*this is where I was crying...oh I was sooooo angry at this point....gosh I hated this hill...here was the Strawberry Lady with THOSE strawberries*! But then I had a totally unexpected reaction. There were big chunks of places, sceneries, areas, that I don't recall at all (probably because I was crying/angry/tuned out). I had a long talk with myself and decided that if I was going to enjoy this more than last time and not have Big Sur kick my butt, I HAD to take in the scenery. Look around at the Red Woods... the ocean..... the cows that were running up and over the hill chasing the runners...Yes! This really happened this year and one of my fondest memories (Tara 3, Big Sur 1).

Back to race day, Rebecca and I had planned to start the race with the 4:30 pace group and see what happened. What happened was we ran with them, or slightly ahead of them, until around mile 9...when they decided to leave us (how dare they). This was right before starting the climb up to Hurricane

Point. But who needs a pace group, when we had each other...and with Rebecca's mountain running hutzpah...we RAN all the way up to Hurricane Point (have I mentioned that to get to Hurricane Point you have to run 2 miles up a 5% grade???). It was not fast and it definitely was not pretty, but we got it done and we got it done with NO tears!!! (Tara 4, Big Sur 1).

Although I am very proud of myself for running all the way up (I walked most of the way last time...with tears), running the whole way may have been the breaking point for Rebecca's hip and my.....nope not my right hamstring, my LEFT IT band...go figure! Shortly after crossing the Bixby Bridge, the official halfway point, Rebecca and I were contemplating taking short walk breaks....I was all for walking because by then the downhills started to kill my IT band. The lofty dream of finishing in 4:30 was over (Tara 4, Big Sur 2). BUT as I kept telling Rebecca, my head was still good. I was still having a great time and if we had to walk the rest of the race I was fine with that. (Tara 5, Big Sur 2).

I do have to say, only because I made a point of mentioning that the Strawberry Lady's strawberries were not all they were cracked up to be last time (for me), the oranges at the Aid Stations were the BEST oranges that I have ever had....ever (Tara 6, Big Sur 2). And the strawberries were pretty great too! And here is also where I have to say that the volunteers for this race are amazingly wonderful. They have to be up and at 'em just as early as we do in order to get on the course before it closes. And they are all very cheery and happy to see us. I cannot say enough about the volunteers and the Big Sur community! I <3 Big Sur (Tara 7 Big Sur 2).

I don't remember exactly when, but things started to go downhill, quickly...and I don't mean in elevation....my IT band was trying it's hardest to get me out of the game. There was more and more walking and the running was getting harder and harder to enjoy. My head was still in the game but it was taking all my energy to convince myself I was having a good time. The finish line is all we wanted to see (Tara 7, Big Sur 3).

And as unbelievable as it seemed...after 26 miles there it was!!! The finish line was in sight!!! The pain was still there, but you can do anything for .2 miles. Right??? I had to convince Rebecca of this, and after 26.1 miles she told me if I felt like it to go ahead. That was NOT going to happen. We started this together 9 months ago, we were going to finish it together!!! And we did... a little worse for wear, but it was DONE!

Want to know something? Even though Big Sur tried it's damnedest, I finished the race with a smile on my face and NO TEARS (Tara 8, Big Sur 3)! AND a new Big Sur PR of 4:54:28 (Tara 9, Big Sur 3). I met 3 out of my 5 goals...not too shabby, if I do say so myself.

Two years ago I became a marathoner (a Big Sur Marathoner). One month ago I went back to kick Big Sur's butt...my score card says.....I got this!!!!!

Training Is Hard, But Oh So Rewarding
By Sheila Dawe

Isn't it funny how when one first gets a new training program there is a wistful dream like quality to imagining conquering all those distances? Yet when the actual training days come there is the cold truth of fear and dread of facing the distance. During the workout, there can be moments of doubt, thoughts of quitting or questioning of one's physical ability. After the workout there is a strong sense of accomplishment, and hope that the next workout will be even more successful.

This year I discovered a very unique training program for my 100 mile ultra. It is by Jeff Galloway and consists of doing 4 "runs" with no longer than 4 hours between each workout. The workouts are every 3-4 weeks with minimal miles in the weekends between, thus allowing for full recovery. In his book he often stresses to walk as much as necessary and on any given run it is still okay to walk the whole thing as you will still gain endurance.

Recently I attempted my greatest distance to date, 85 miles. Here is a little glimpse of an ultra-training weekend:

Friday, May 15th: 7:30 pm – I lay down dressed in my running outfit, hoping for a little sleep before I start my training at 10:45 tonight. I listen to the sound of kids playing, dogs barking and tell myself, any rest is good for my body, even if I don't actually fall asleep. 10:00 pm. Perhaps I should get up. 10:30 pm. I am wakened by my alarm. Odd how sometimes the thought of getting up and not trying to sleep results in a release and sleep finally finding me.

Run 1 – 10:45 pm to 4:15 am. I am out the door. It is 16 C and I head off to a road which will take me above our town. As usual the start is tough, as it is so daunting the distance and time you will still have to cover. I reflect back to the beginning of my program when I only did 5 miles for the first run, today I am to go the farthest yet with 20 miles. I little bit of the adventurer in me is excited to see how far along Nanaimo Lakes Road this will take me. I pass through a small park where bats dart in and out of my vision when I look up, scanning the trees for fear of Cougars. Thankfully no cat eyes are reflected back and all I see are lots of killer bunny rabbits and hear various choruses of frogs.

Run 2 – 7:30 am to 1:30 pm. Saturday, May 16th. After a very brief lay down, I was up again and ready to go…sort of. My first run was with my mother, we did a gentle 4 mile route. Then she drove home and I ran the 14 mile route we had done together in her training for her half marathon. About half way I stopped at a rest area, sat at a picnic bench and laid down my head. I was so tired, I could go to sleep BUT that would not get me home or get my training done. I finished the route and then walked the 3 miles home for a total distance of 21 miles.

Run 3 – 5:00 pm to 12:10 am. It is still a lovely day but this would be a tricky one as the evening would be in full swing by the time I finish – tricky to dress for such changes in the temperature. I am now in full on walk mode but keeping myself motivated for this 24 mile adventure. I listened to several audible books and really enjoyed getting lost in the world of Science Fantasy. I visited 7-11 twice for refueling. On the return walk I sat at a bus stop bench while I ate some food. I focused on how many miles left to get home, I translate this into time left which I find easier to mentally deal with when I am getting tired…so only 2 more hours. When I got up my shins tightened up so much it really hurt to walk. However after a few steps, they loosened up and I was fine, that is until I got home and had to face a flight of stairs. I set my alarm for 3:30 am and mentally was questioning whether I would be able to do the fourth run.

Run 4 – 4:10 am to 6:40 am Sunday, May 17th. Slow, slow as molasses, slow as a slug – is this really worth it. It is time for some serious self-talk. I was supposed to do 21 miles, perhaps if I could just go out 6 miles. As I continued on it then changed to "just get to 5 miles". But at 4 miles, I thought "nope, this is all I got, I best turn around". Funny thing happened on the return trip – I began to feel good. I even ran a slow single mile to keep my running streak days alive. I came up with all sorts of plans, as I wasn't completing my scheduled distance – doing only 8 miles for my final run resulted in a total of 73 miles instead of 85 miles.

The next day I felt very good and recovered well. I questioned whether I pushed myself hard enough or whether I should have gone further. But I know that it is better to end feeling good versus having the wheels fall off or worst becoming injured. I have a new plan for the remaining training sessions. Yes, it will be hard but I am sure with all these struggles not only am I gaining physical endurance but I am also gaining mental endurance. I think that the more barriers I push through, the more I will gain come that day in September. With each and every training session, I think I always gain a little bit more knowledge of who I am and what I am capable of. Keep on keeping on.

Training is hard and yet can also be very gratifying. There are no race day photos, no bib, no expo, no aid stations, no cheering spectators, no start time, and no medal at the end. But if you put in the miles, embrace the workout; then you will be rewarded on race day.

Every Mile Matters
By Elaine Knipe

As a middle school kid, I got the opportunity to run track. As I ran three years of track, what I enjoyed the most was being competitive and running fast. I must admit I hated any track event with any long distance and why well because I wanted the fast and quick results at that time in my running. That's the runners high I was after. Unfortunately, after middle school my running diminished and the zeal for running was forgotten about. I no longer looked for the satisfaction of running which I look back now with regret. Moving forward 11 years, mid-twenties with a struggle of addiction on my hands and needing some sort of release and way to cope of how to get my life right. Running was coming up in my head to pick back up, and so I did and with every time I went out the door to run. My head and heart was starting to know of what I needed to start to do.

As I was getting situated in this new clean lifestyle running was back in my life. My runs weren't with any real long distance but enough to be part of the much needed therapy that my life needed. Almost every day a 30 min run was part of my day first thing. With completion of treatment and laying out of what's next in this rebuilding of my life, the constant hustle and bustle of life which entailed the finding of clean and sober living, finding of a sponsor, work and striving of how to be reunited with my children who were living with my parents as I went and got treatment. Yet again at this time in my life running took back burner and diminished. What was I thinking? I don't know but again look back with regret on why this activity that I knew that added to my happiness was on the way side.

For years it remained this way, I forgot the awesomeness of running and the therapy that it gave me. Being established in my life and raising my children and now married I had become overweight and was not active in any way except for work and caring for my family. We had signed onto a gym membership in our area and used it maybe once, twice a week. Then friends we had just met also had signed up for a membership and come to find out she was a runner. With it being years of not hearing that word running, it was like walking past an old friend that you were pleased to see again. At this point I almost forgot how to start or even know what to do .However; I was soon reunited to my old friend running. She asked me if I wanted to start running with her in the mornings before our families woke up. With feeling of hesitation and excitement I did it! Up at 4:30 and running at 5 am I was on a treadmill. Ready but nervous I pushed "go" on the treadmill and it was time to get to it, let's do this and see where it goes this time.

After doing 2 miles I felt as if I completed the Boston Marathon, what an accomplishment with being overweight and unhealthy. Wanted to quit that whole week, but I knew I needed to stick it out. Then she said," Lets run outside 4 miles on Sat Morning." With immediately feeling a lack of confidence, to be able to complete, I pushed on anyway. I said, "I would be there." Saturday came and it was early morning with the sky of pretty pink and blue and sun starting to rise and the cool just right tempts and the quietness that you get to have when you get up crazy early .It was like the town belonged only to us. So we parked at the gym and started to head to a scenic part of Sandy. Yikes! My lungs and legs started to burn not far from where we started and I was thinking to myself what happened to my love for running? My feelings of hating what I was doing was confusing me and had me discouraged but kept going with stop and walk and then run again method. I just couldn't wait for the next break to come. As we pass the scenic view of the beauty before us was when I started to appreciate the pain I was going through and running wasn't an enemy but rather a friend I had to get to know again and wanted too. As we headed to the end of our run, it was bittersweet, I wanted to continue but my body was saying leave it for another day. I hugged her and thanked her over and over for getting me out and getting me reacquainted to running again. As the week went on there were days she couldn't meet but I would go anyway on my own. It was an opportunity for me to see what I was going to do with this. I was running 3-4 times a week, before

I knew it and loved it. Couldn't wait for the next time I could run. Again it was my therapy, my chance to think, to challenge myself. In no time I was running 5 miles, 7 miles, 10 miles and being someone who hated long distance I sure loved my long run days. Today, running is my challenge to myself that I constantly keep reevaluating. First, it was to be fast and win, then distance to cover and now it's to do long distance and speed. My goal is to run Boston one day and will keep striving until I do. And that is what running has taught me is to keep striving in all aspects of my life. The extra special blessing that running has given me I get to at times run with my kids and hubby they will go on runs with me, do races with me and will support me in my running. Even though running has been in and out of my life it has given me what I have needed at that time, for that I am forever grateful.

Every Mile Matters – Know Why It Matters to YOU
By Melissa Oltman

I didn't start running until I was 53 years old – in fact, I made it a point to tell people that I didn't run, and I had no interest in running. Ever. The truth was, I had been interested a few times in my life; once in high school, when I couldn't run the required mile to qualify for the gymnastics team, and once in the 1980's, when Jim Fixx was all the rage with his running book. I had tried to run, and I sucked at it.

But in September 2013 I WALKED a 5K at my new job, and something clicked. The people who had run looked like they had so much fun, and I wanted to feel that! So the following Monday I started the Couch to 5K app. And by Friday I had strained the medial meniscus on both knees and could hardly walk! I honestly don't know what made me keep trying. Certainly, I had given up before, but SOMETHING stuck with me.

By January I had found Moon Joggers, and I wanted what THOSE people had too: the joy, the friendships, the fun at races. To make a long story short, I entered my first half marathon because "Of course you can!" from my favorite enabler and cheerleader Carolyn. It was the Chicago Rock and Roll Half Marathon, July 20, 2014. I was all flustered when my GPS wouldn't work amidst the tall buildings of Chicago, so I couldn't tell if I was keeping the right pace, so I finally just forgot about it and PRANCED my way through 13 glorious miles! It got tough that last mile – man, it was tough! But I finished on the highest high I have ever felt in my life! I could easily have turned right around and run the whole thing again.

And that's really when things went sour. I raced again in August, and again in September – oh, THAT one was wonderful. A whole BUNCH of Moon Joggers met in Dayton, Ohio for the Air Force Marathon, and you have never really RUN until you have run with a whole bunch of people who have become friends, comrades, and teammates. I actually got really sick at that one – heat exhaustion – because I had gone out too fast, and barely limped across the finish line before being hauled into the medic tent with low blood pressure. See, I had fallen prey to the "What's your pace?" monster. They say that "comparison is the thief of joy" and as the months progressed, comparing myself to everyone else slowly poisoned what had become for me not only one of my greatest joys but definitely my stress reliever. Indeed, running became MORE stressful, as I would look down at that bloody Garmin 50 times during each run, and how I felt was totally dependent on that "average pace per mile" flashing on my wrist.

I ran in October and in December – I actually really loved the December race, but I didn't sign up for any halfs after that because I noticed that not only was I comparing myself to others, but there was a sneaky little thing, even among friends, of comparing themselves to me and amongst each other.

I ran my first marathon in Little Rock on March 1, 2015, and unfortunately, I became injured on my last long run 4 weeks out from it, so the experience itself was painful and disappointing. There was so much I LOVED about it. The city itself is wonderful, the sights we passed were incredible, and the people you meet in those last 6 miles and the conversations you have are very cool, but my time goal was impossible because of my injury.

And when I finished I honestly didn't care if I ever ran again. At first I thought it was normal – most people take time off after a marathon because the training can be pretty consuming. But I just couldn't get it back. I tried a lot of things. I tried the positive self talk, the switching up cross training. I tried it all, but for me, the thrill was very much gone. And I really really grieved that. Running has been so many things for me.

And then recently, a very smart and wise friend told me, "Stop trying so hard.

Don't wear your Garmin, don't log your miles. Just get out the door and go." And one early morning, all by myself, I stepped out the door – no Garmin, no nothing, and just took off down the street with no real plan of where I was running or for how far or how long. And about half a block into it, I was very aware of my shoulders relaxing, and I closed my eyes and took a deep breath and just sighed. Because it just felt SO GOOD to be out there doing MY thing all by myself.

Find out why every mile matters TO YOU PERSONALLY. There's nothing wrong with wanting to be faster, but for me, personally, I am very much NOT a competitive person. It's my hippie-everyone-wins personality. For me, running is my ME time, the one time in the day when I am not responsible for anyone else, I have no decisions to make except whether to turn right or turn left, and I am the most authentically Melissa. I love to do races for the FUN – it's like going to a big party, for me. And I have finally learned to not only be OK with all of that, but to stand up for it, and hold tightly to it when others have different goals and needs.

Every single blessed mile matters to ME. It's MINE – my experience, my achievement, on my terms. And I truly hope that every runner finds out and cherishes why every mile matters to THEM.

Every Mile Matters
by V. Kowalewski

I was a competitive 3-sport jock in high school, but I hated running. HATED.
IT. Many years and several pounds later I decided I'd take up running as a way
to get in shape and lose some weight. My first run was to a small bridge over a
creek ½ mile away from my house. I SERIOUSLY thought I was going to die
before I got to the end of the block, and I was pretty sure that bridge was
getting further away instead of closer.

That experience was humbling to say the least. It hurt my pride and kinda
pissed me off. So I signed up for the Bellringer 5 mile run in my hometown
over 4th of July. They had a 2 mile, but hey where's the challenge. I did the 5.
And peed myself halfway through. And poured water from the water stations
down my front hoping to camouflage the fact that I had just run so hard I'd
lost control of my bladder yet was one of the last to finish.

In the 20+ years since that "run" to the bridge things have changed a lot. I've
done distances from 5K up to Marathon and events ranging from obstacle and
snowshoe races to trail runs and Ragnar relay. I've raced in a barbarian
costume and a tutu. TWICE. When I'm not training for an event I'm still
running just because I enjoy it. Running brings a few minutes of peace to a
chaotic existence. Problems seem easier to solve when I'm on a run.

These feet have seen a lot of miles in the 20+ years since that first run and I
would have to say without a doubt every last one of them served a purpose.
Miles for strength. Miles to challenge myself. Miles running away from grief
and stress. Miles to purge despair and emptiness. Miles for peace and

harmony. Miles for new adventures and experience. Miles to celebrate being alive. Miles to just BE BETTER.

Running's certainly been an unlimited source of goals to chase. This year I'm coming back from an unexpected setback and the goal is to see if I can run various distances faster than last year, maybe faster than EVER. So far I'm doing pretty well with that, and it's been a blast! I've also been doing events with other people for fun instead of time. After years of running alone, it's weird to do something like Ragnar with a team that's counting on you to perform or Warrior Dash with people who don't give a care and just want to have fun, or just going to a regular road race with a friend.

As I've grown older the focus definitely has become more about just challenging myself and enjoying the absolute snot out of the journey. These days I treasure every mile I'm able to put in. Time is precious and every mile has meaning. They're not all glorious and effortless, but they're not all suffering and toil either. It is what it is, and right now it's GOOD.

Why do I run? Because life truly is a gift, and of all the things I do to stay as healthy as possible so that I can ENJOY the gift running is what makes me feel the most....ALIVE. Thanks, running friends, for all your support and encouragement on this amazing journey!

———————

V. Kowalewski is an Organizational Knowledge Analyst currently enjoying living, running and crocheting in the great 4-season state of MN and anywhere else she can manage to get to and do the same. She thinks cheese and craft beers are pretty awesome too.

Every Mile Matters
By Lisa Ledman

I ran for healing.
In 2010, my world, as I knew it, seemed to be falling apart all around me. Five people in my family were fighting Cancer, I lost the job I loved, and my overall health was at an all-time low. Loss was all around me and I felt consumed by it. I started looking for a way out of the darkness. I began this journey by getting up each morning to read my bible, pray and reflect. During this time of reflection I was observing how my friend Veronica had changed her health by taking action and running and so it began. I took baby steps...started out by doing walk/run intervals and slowly worked up to running 3 miles. At this time in my life I ran for healing.

I ran for fitness.
In 2013, I wanted to improve my fitness level and heal physically – I was now 49 and the milestone of turning 50 was looming. This goal required accountability, consistency, and a plan as I was still carrying a surplus of 50 lbs on my frame. My friends, Stacy and Veronica, pointed me in the right direction. Stacy encouraged me to start a 10-week Challenge at Farrell's Extreme Body Shaping gym, which focused on nutrition, strength-training, and cardio through kickboxing. During this 10-week period I continued to run and lost 20 lbs and a total of 20.5 inches off my frame. It felt so good and I had learned what I needed to do. Veronica told me about Moon Joggers and I decided to give it a try. Moon Joggers provided the accountability and encouragement to train and run my first races – some 5Ks and 10Ks. This accountability worked and I lost an additional 20 lbs and felt amazing when I turned 50 in May of 2014. At this time in my life I ran for fitness.

I ran for enjoyment.

In 2014, I wanted to run for fun! I felt amazing and really loved running races. I loved it all, the training, the outfits, the adrenaline rush, the food, the beverages, the comradery and of course the medals! Through encouragement from my Moon Jogger virtual friends (especially Calla and Carolyn) and Veronica I signed up for my first half-marathon, Whistlestop, in Ashland, Wisconsin. My daughter, Kristi and cousin, Andy came with to cheer me on and I had the most amazing time. I had the race bug! I signed up for lots of races which included 5Ks, 10Ks, 15Ks, snow-shoe races, trail runs, and obstacle courses and set out on a new goal to reach Half-Fanatics status. This past Sunday, I reached this goal at the Chicago Rock and Roll Half Marathon and I enjoyed every minute of this trip. At this time in my life I ran for enjoyment.

The reasons I run have changed with the seasons of my life. More than anything I have realized that "Every Mile Matters" to my mind, body, and soul – I run for me! As of today, I am not sure what will drive me to continue to run in 2015 or beyond; but I know I will continue. I will continue to run for healing, fitness, and pure enjoyment.

Every Mile Matters
By Laura Lok

Hi my name is Laura Lok from Spokane, Washington.   I started my adventure with running like many do late in life and for a reason. Mine was for a friend that wanted to join Team In Training to raise money in support of her sister in law that was battling leukemia. I said "I will do it with you." She didn't even ask but a pair is always better than one and helps motivate each other. It went well and I walked my first half marathon at the Nike Women's half in San Francisco. Everyone thought I was nuts to walk that far and prior to the event the most I had done was 10 miles. I cried at mile 11. Received my bling and crashed for a few hours afterwards.

I never thought I would do it again. Just a one time bucket list kind of thing

WRONG

Something happened as I crossed that finish line and I picked up my medal, I fell in love with the race. The people I met along the way. The fact that I could actually accomplish this after a couple of months of training. The finisher shirt, the medal. All of it.

So I continued a few more races walking mostly with an occasional jog usually near the end.

After about 2 years I started running a bit more but always became winded. My legs could go for miles but not my lungs. The doc says I have reactive airway disease. Whatever I thought he made that up, yeah I know they don't make things up. I started an inhaler and things were better but not great.

This past year I started running more than walking. The more I go the better I get. Imagine that TRAINING really is training your body to handle it better and better. I still only run once or twice a week but the rest of the week I get in lots of walking or hiking. When training for a half I increase my running to 3 times a week with a long run but sometimes walk at a very fast pace on the weekend. I think that combo has really helped me do better. At almost 50 and on my 13th official half I finally achieved my goal of a 2:30 half. Yeah I am no speed demon but if I keep this up I may eventually get to 2:00 someday. But if not oh well, I'll keep at it. The races have taken me all over. Giving me an excuse for a girl's weekend or mini trip.

I have 3 more halves to do this year, all with friends and mostly hilly or destinations like Las Vegas. Not expecting to beat that time because these races are about friendship. I have friends that are faster and some that are slower we each go with what we feel like for the day. One of the reasons races mean so much to me is the people. My friends and people I met along the way and hear their story.

I have had people say you have been my rat this race thank you for helping me keep a pace and not give up. The last 3 miles of one race a gal I started talking with said it was her first race and she had never done more than 8 miles she didn't think she was going to make it. We talked some more and another mile gone and another finally I said "You know you have only half a mile left you got this." She thanked me and said she couldn't have done it without me. She could have she just needed another reason to keep going and I was there to be that reason. You never know who you will inspire as a slow runner or a fast runner. We are all out there making our miles count for a reason, whether we know the reason yet or not.

Run or walk for your health or for a cause every step you take takes you someplace you haven't been before.

Fat Girls Can Run, Too
By Christina Leeper

On August 11, 2014, my life changed FOREVER. The emergency room doctor looked me in the eye and said, "Mrs. Leeper, you are going to be dead by Christmas if you don't do something NOW. I don't want to upset you, but that is the reality that we are facing." For once in my life, I was speechless.

I was 44 years old at the time....obese....smoking over a pack a day....diabetes out of control....let's face it, folks: I was a hot mess. I was that person that NEVER went to the doctor. I rationalized that I didn't "have time" to exercise and I definitely "couldn't afford" to eat healthy. I was plagued with "not feeling well" just about all the time – so much so that I actually didn't notice that it was becoming nearly a constant thing. Then, on August 11, 2014, I was at work and I REALLY felt bad. I told my manager I was going to drive myself to the Emergency Room. When I got there, they took me to the little triage room to check my vital signs. The automated blood pressure machine started beeping, and the sweet girl who was typing in the numbers looked up. I watched all the color drain from her face as she tried to control her voice. "Mrs. Leeper," she said, "I am going to be right back." Then, she bolted from the room. Confused, I looked up to see what my blood pressure was. The screen said it was 242/212.

Two days later I went to my new partner in wellness, Martha Fletcher (she's awesome, by the way, as is everyone at my doctor's office). Not only was my blood pressure was out of control....my A1C (long-term measurement of blood sugar) was 11 (it's supposed to be under 7). I should weigh around 135-165 –

my weight that day was 280 pounds. I couldn't walk one flight of stairs without wheezing. Martha said I needed to get it together. I cried a lot. But we made a plan, and I got it together.

I started walking on a treadmill for 30 minutes a day, three days a week. I was really surprised at how fast my body got used to the exercise….I moved it to 4 days a week. Then I started increasing the speed of the treadmill, and then the incline. And then one day, I realized that I could not progress any more just walking. *IT WAS TIME TO RUN.*

I have been obese just about my entire adult life. I could spend a lot of time talking about why – let's just say I am someone who enjoys eating my feelings, which makes me feel bad about myself, so I just eat more. But I had a secret dream, one that I hadn't told anyone, not even my family: I wanted to run. It looked like so much fun! But Fat Girls Can't Run, right? That is what I believed for over 20 years. Fat. Girls. Can't. Run. So here I am, walking on the treadmill, and I realize I was about to run. First lesson that I learned about running. I HATE RUNNING ON THE TREADMILL.

I made a daring decision. I was going to run outside. Where people could see me. I had heart palpitations just considering it. So, I started running REALLY early in the morning. It was still dark, and the only other people out were other runners. Nobody would see me. BONUS: Sunrise is a beautiful time of day to be outside. I started using a Couch-to-5K app and did jog/walk intervals. 30 minutes, three days a week. I was hooked. I got my first pair of Brooks. I got my first knee brace. I got my first armband to hold my phone. Lesson learned: SHOPPING FOR RUNNING STUFF IS FUN.

Then, I discovered Moon Joggers. What an amazing community! I learned many lessons very quickly – such as "If you are going faster than a walk, then you are a RUNNER." Whoo-hoo! I was a runner! I started running in the daylight. Other runners would smile at me and say hi, or give me a high-five as we passed each other on the trail. Holy cow, this is FUN!!!

I ran my first 5K. I discovered virtual races. Lesson learned: YOU GET COOL MEDALS IF YOU RUN VIRTUAL RACES. Medals are FUN. I love my bling!

Oh, by the way, I lost 59 pounds, and did my first 10K in March. Then life happened, and I had to quit running for a while. I've gained back 20 pounds. But I haven't given up. Because #FatGirlsCanRunToo – and I will always be a runner. I may have to start my C25K over again. I may have to haul out the knee brace. But, dammit, I am going to be back in my skinny jeans by the time cold weather hits, because I know how good it feels, and I want that feeling back. The moral of the story: Nike had it right….you have to Just Do It. Don't think about it, don't make excuses. Get off the couch and walk for 30 minutes. Keep doing that until you know it is time to take it to the next level. Then pick up the pace and run. It's amazing. It's the best thing that ever happened to me. Let it be the best thing that happens to you, too.

Why I Keep Movin'
Every Mile Matters
by Val

This isn't one of those heart-string-tugging stories. Nor is it a bittersweet journey of learning about running or who I am. It is just a simple story of two girls who got me moving, a family that believes I am strong and a lost son. And maybe why I keep movin'.

The two ladies on either side of me are my two younger sisters – they are runners !!! They were going with a group to Florida for the 20th Anniversary WDW Marathon in 2013. So why couldn't I go? Because I am 50 lbs. over weight, I smoke, I walk, I don't run ! Top 3 reasons to not even think about doing something as silly as trying to attempt a marathon. Those girls trained and trained...and so did I for the next 8 months. I lost 20 lbs., quit smoking in public (yes, I would "sneak" a couple every couple of days if I'm going to be honest) and I walked, then slowly jogged, then walked some more. My feet hurt, my legs hurt and my back hurt, no matter how much I walked. But I pressed on. They all live in Michigan, I live in Northern California. Can you already guess what the temperature difference is going to be for all of us?

As I said above these two girls are runners so they could have started in one of the earlier starting corrals. They opted to stay with me in the middle of the last corral. I felt special and Blessed to have these ladies sticking with me. We were together until the start line then they took off at their own pace. I didn't see them again till we all gathered around the finish. They both finished and I was (still am) very proud of them, it was their first marathon. I made it to 14 miles when the heat finally caught up with me and I threw in the towel and took the bus to the finish line. I said that day that I would never do another race.

Those girls have kept me inspired. I have since done 5 half marathons. I did the Humboldt Bay Inaugural Marathon/Half Marathon a couple of weeks ago and although I finished it wasn't pretty. I had some terrible personal issues slam me to the ground 4 months ago...my son died very unexpectedly at the age of 42 in April of this year. I did a half in May in honor of him and I have to admit it was good therapy and a decent time (3:25). I kept moving and finished in my best time ever with loads of encouragement from friends along the way. But from that day to the day of the Humboldt Bay Run I haven't put my shoes on except for one attempt. Everything seems to bring me down, the river I walk beside, the birds in the trees, the cows in the pasture. Why should the world go on? That run took me just shy of 4 hours, my feet hurt, my legs hurt and I got dehydrated. I tried every way I could think of to talk myself into just sitting down and waiting for the wagon to pick me up. But you see, as everyone who knows me will tell you, I am not a quitter. I am strong. My brother calls me the Rock of the family (they are all my biggest supporters and strength). And I don't give up easily. So I straightened my backbone, dug for a little more determination, thought of my son and happy times, and cried my way to the finish line. With only half a dozen people behind me it was finished. And I smiled. I know he would be proud of me for finishing.

I am now signed up for another half in October and am determined to get back to my 3:15 (3:30) walking speed. Thanks to my sisters for all your encouragement. Thanks to local friends for their support. And thanks to Moon Joggers who daily inspire me.
–VAL

I Will Be THAT Girl
By Linda Hodges

I know I'm late writing my article but I'll explain why in a bit. First let me apologize in advance for misspelled words, very poor grammar and well my horrific writing skills (I was that C-D grammar student). Now with that said here we go.

I'm not sure if you know anything about me, so let me introduce myself! My name is Linda, I'm a 43 year old married, mother of 4, grandmother of 5 (#6 due anytime). I'm a disabled registered nurse, former bookstore owner, electronic geek and many more titles. The thing is most people who see me these days see me as the unconventional uncontrolled diabetic, past CVA chick (brain attacks, stroke) in 2011 & 2013, past MI (heart attack) with stent placement January 2015, severe neuropathy girl, and now the super depressed obese lady.

For most my life I've allowed my diagnosis dictate who or what I was. I allowed all the doctors to use medical terms to describe me, and I sat quietly while others determined what my life would look like. There has been days I'm tired of being sick and tired. I have suffered from depression so badly that I have stayed in bed, binged ate till my glucose wouldn't measure on home machines and cried thru out my showers. Depression paralyzed me and stole all my joy. It prevented me from completing anything including this story. I also gained a whopping 85 lbs in a year, this year to be on point. I tell you this to say….I'm over this, I don't want to be THAT girl anymore.

As a teen I ran track, long distance was my favorite. I loved getting into that perfect pace and letting every care I had slip under my feet. I looked forward to that shaky adrenaline filled person I became after a good run. Then as I became older with kids I looked forward to long walks pushing my rug rats in strollers. Now.....well now life is different I have days I can barely feel my feet thanks to neuropathy, my right side is weak from the strokes, and my heart thinks I'm in a marathon every time I check the mail. There is days I need to use an aide to walk, I have canes, standard walker, rolling walker, a wheel chair and an electric wheel chair. And again I don't want to be THAT girl anymore.

The one thing I didn't mention I am a Moon Jogger! I joined on the maiden trip to the moon.   Thanks to my most popular very pretty cousin Carolyn Guhman. I was introduced to some wild and crazy folks. I instantly fell back in love with a life that I could no longer have, but was accepted anyway. As some ran marathons, I struggled to get in my 5k after an entire week but I was still accepted. I have NEVER met any of my goals and that is OK. I set more and moved on. Even with your acceptance I was too embarrassed to mention how deeply the darkness had become...I didn't want to be THAT girl.

So here I sat feeling all kinds of blue all in my emotions. It was the one of the constants in my life. Wake up take meds, check my blood sugar, adjust my insulin pump watch TV, let the darkness control me, go to sleep...repeat. Till I became tired of THAT girl. This hasn't been months ago but rather last week. So I have no wonderful results to share but I want to throw this out there into the universe for all to read. I'm done with THAT girl!!!

I can't give you that exact ah ha moment, maybe it was several tiny moments. I literally woke up last week, looked in the mirror and was in shock at what I saw...in front of me was a broken person. Darkened eyes, hair was a nappy mess, and the weight I had gained so quickly has left me wearing very unflattering clothing from my mothers closet. Yes a loving woman she is but never known for her stylish qualities. I defiantly don't want to be THAT girl in the mirror any more.

Thank goodness for strong relationships I have in my life. As a nurse we were taught depression can destroy everything a person holds dear. My husband is a rock, he has taken everything with the strength unlike I've ever seen. His love has been proven over and over because it had to be love and faith that has kept him from running. From the reflection in the mirror anyone else would have ran for the hills. I told him a few nights ago that I was tired and ready to be happy. You know what he said, I kid you not he said "that's my girl". Now I must say I wanna be THAT girl!

Everyone of you are so very dear to me, I read your struggles, I celebrate your successes and I pray for you daily. I wait to hear of your results from races, your last doctor appointment from an injury and I'm so excited when you get the all clear to hit the road. When Perry ran across the US I became so fixated that I felt as though I was with him as he ran...THANK YOU PERRY! So know your post are being enjoyed. (Keep posting)

So in the past week I've joined a gym, been swimming once, and started a Tai Chi class. Tomorrow is a huge day because I'll start on a treadmill. I'm going to take this "every mile matters" slogan to a new level. I might even measure the distance should I fall, that should count just unsure on the equation I should use. I'm excited again.

Tonight while I stood in line (unassisted) at the drug store, I received a message from our fearless leader, Angie. She was letting me know how well the phone home ET themed virtual run had turned out. I had been so depressed that I barely even acknowledged that y'all had a virtual race in my honor. THANK YOU!! I promise to fight the dark clouds, to lose the weight and be the best possible me regardless of my health. I will be THAT girl!

EVERY MILE MATTERS....
by Harmony Drogosz

We all want to achieve our goals with those who mean the most to us. There are many milestones, hardships and victories with each goal completion. Every story encourages another to do their best, to have fun and to be inspired. Running was all of this to me. Why? Because you can push the limits! My achievements have been successful because I was inspired by my best friend who got me to be passionate about running, to start small and to finish with your best. We signed up for our first race almost 3 years ago after training to reach our 3 mile marker. And to our surprise we gathered a great support group that included our significant others, my kids, and my bestie's boyfriend's father. They all watched us from the start line, walked throughout the course to watch our progress and headed over to the finish line to watch us complete the race. The whole race, the vibe, the cheering from the people we love most was exhilarating.

That winter my husband got a better job and we were separated by a 13 hour drive. Our will to continue to run and to find races didn't end. We traveled together so we can race, make faster times, run longer distances as a team. My family didn't travel with me as often as I wanted but I still had their support and thanks to my best friend she always had her family (husband and father-in-law) to cheer us on. Distance was nothing to us considering everything we trained for, keeping the same pace, her wedding, and more races. Everything that we were a part of had her father-in-law right there to support us. Our 30k race was her father-in-law's last one with us. Even though he was ill he was there at the finish line for us cheering us on. Still the loving, caring man he always was. This was a rough time for us since he couldn't be there for her first wedding anniversary.

Needless to say our next race was the full on marathon, when we arrived to check in our bags, the details he kept away from us was all there, right in front of us. The UPS truck, the last name, and the day he died was on that truck. We knew he was with us, still giving us all his support. Throughout the course when we thought about giving up, a UPS truck was there and we were inspired to keep running and we made it to the finish line knowing he was our encouragement through the hard times, the reason our milestones were so amazing and why our victories were honorable! In the upcoming months we will continue to run his last race on a yearly basis as a monument of a man who loved us, inspired us, believed in us and who taught of the true meanings of life. Even though the miles were never counted by us, to him every mile mattered!

If at first you don't succeed...try...try...and try again
By Sheila Dawe

In 2010 I completed my first 100 km event in Lethbridge, Alberta at a race called Lost Souls Ultra. I registered in early January and then in mid-March fell on some stairs, tearing a tendon in my knee. I went through physiotherapy and had about 6 months to recover. In hind sight I think this was a blessing as my first 100 km was a pure walk due to the instability of my knee. LSU is a hilly course (my first year with sore knees I did every downhill backwards). It has 3 distances: 53 km, 100 km, and 100 mile. The 100 km and 100 mile start on the Friday 8 am and racers have to finish by Saturday evening at 7 pm, giving them 35 hours to complete. The 53 km starts Saturday morning at 7 am, giving racers 12 hours to complete.

There are 3 aid stations on the course (Headquarters, Peemaquin, and Pavan), the racers do a 53 km or 33 mile loop, and arrive at these aid stations both from a North and South directions, depending how far they are into the loop. In my first year, I remember being at my penultimate aid station, Peemaquin, on the second morning and seeing a 100 mile competitor heading out for his 3rd and final 53 km lap. I looked at him with awe and thought to myself that someday that that could be me. However, I knew that I would need to get faster to have enough time.

In 2011 and 2012, I repeated the 100 km distances. Each year, as my knees improve, I would run a little bit more and improve my finish time: 2010 – 26:48, 2011 – 24:18 and 2012 – 21:39. Finally in 2013 I decided to go for the

100 mile distance. LSU used to give out finisher rocks but in 2013 they changed to giving rocks only to those that placed in their age category. Not many women finished the 100 mile and in fact the year I decided to move up to the 100 mile distance there were no female 50+ age finishers. I felt that if I could finish it would be very likely that I would place and get a coveted rock, turns out that was a very big IF.

Wanting, trying, pushing oneself becomes unimaginably hard on the second morning of an ultra. In both in 2013 and 2014, despite having enough time, I mentally convinced myself I was too slow and dropped out at the 82 mile mark. This year I was convinced it would be different. I had trained harder, starting in December, culminating with 4 weekends over the summer where I put in 73 plus miles. I felt ready. In addition I had a great pacer lined up (he would join me for the 3rd and final loop). He had specific instructions to deal with my mind and try to not let me quit. I had given him some key phrases and tried to focus on wanting to share the course with someone else. Knowing that you are going to have company and moral support is priceless and keeps the ultra-runner/walker motivated through the night to get to their final lap and have their pacer join them.

I never imagined that this year it would be as hot as it turned out to be. Unfortunately I was not acclimated coming from cooler B.C. climate and visiting the Yukon the week prior. Early on I went into conservation mode and walked far more than I have any other year beside 2010. The result was that I was one hour off my time when I met my pacer. I knew I did not have enough time to get to the first time cut-off. There came a pivotal moment at Peemaquin, day 2. I was in the same position as that first year when I saw that 100 miler, albeit, it was somewhat later in the day. The time keeper came up and informed me of the cut-off time at the next aid station. I stated that I knew the time and knew I would not make it in time but I would still like to continue on the additional 9.6 km to get once again to my 82 mile cut-off point. I wanted to continue on until the race officials told me that I was officially done. So with pacer in tow we headed out to the grueling hot coulees with 5 black diamond hills at my pitifully slow snail's pace.

There was a lot of soul searching in the 3 hours it took me to cover nearly 10 km. There was a moment where I could have taken a short cut, but chose not to. There was the moment when my good friend Natalie on her return and less than 12 km from the finish yelled to me, "I'm sorry" from across the coulees. She knew that once again I would come up 18 miles short of my goal. My pacer and I discussed whether the maximum distance that I am capable of was 82 miles. Should I continue to try at something that seems to be just out of my reach?

The answer came to me immediately the next day. Not only was I presented with a rock from my two good friends who both finished the 100 mile distance. I realized that despite not finishing I enjoyed every moment of the experience. I have made some very deep friendships. I enjoy challenging myself with something that is not a sure thing. I enjoy the scenery and now at this point I truly know that course. I will be back next year because there is one other thing I am sure of...I will never succeed if I don't keep on trying. Keep on keeping on my friends.

Every Mile Matters
By Michele Ridolfi O'Neill

See that photo? That's a photo of me crossing the finish line at the Brooklyn Rock n Roll half marathon last Saturday, October 10. My arms are raised in victory and I'm grinning from ear to ear, but my happiness in this moment doesn't tell you the full story of how I got there or why that finish—or running—means so much to me. Every mile ran in that race and the many races and training runs leading up to it, counts, and we can only run the mile we're in. That's why I decided to write this blog post.

Before I can tell you about my evolution as a runner, I should tell you a little about myself. I was born in Brooklyn, NY, and although I grew up watching the New York City Marathon and running around my backyard, I was never a "Runner". I had enjoyed running relay races as a pre-teen in gym class, but at some point, I started to get slower as running got harder, so I stopped even trying to race, much less caring about it. After my family moved to Connecticut and I became an adult, I toyed with the idea of running for fitness, but by then I'd learned that I'd developed asthma, and since the simple act of running down my parents' street left me winded, I quickly abandoned it and focused on other activities.

Fast forward about 15 years, to 2013. At that time, I was a relatively new mom with a brand-new career and about 30 pounds of leftover baby weight to lose, even though my "baby" at this point was four years old. It was April, and the weather was getting warmer, and his favorite activity was driving his battery-operated car up and down our cul-de-sac. I would walk alongside his car, but I could scarcely keep up with it. One afternoon as I trailed behind him, he called,

"Mommy, run with me!" and reached his hand out for me to hold. I had to run or one of us was going to end up on the pavement, so I kept up with him for as long as I could. To my surprise, I found that I actually enjoyed running with him, and that I could keep up for more time than I expected. To challenge myself while making my son happy, I made a game out of it, saying, "I'll see if I can run up the whole street" and then, "Let me see if I can run up the street and then back down the street". Before I knew it, I had run about a little over a quarter of a mile without stopping. The next day, I went outside without my son, and decided to time myself running. I was able to get to about eight minutes before I got winded and needed to take a walking break. I was really starting to enjoy it.

Then, the Boston Marathon bombing happened. Like so many others, I couldn't understand why anyone would want to harm so many innocent runners and bystanders. The tragedy inspired me to continue running, and around that time, I registered for my first 5k. I had no plan and no idea what I was doing, but I found running more freeing than any exercise I had ever tried, so I did some online research and discovered the "Couch 2 5k" app. I downloaded it and began using it to train in earnest. The quarter mile I started out running quickly increased to a mile, and then two, and within about three months, I had progressed to running a full three miles. It wasn't easy—there were times where I wondered why I was even trying to run when I could barely begin without feeling like I needed to take my rescue inhaler—but there were also wonderful times where my body felt lighter than it had in years and my mind clearer. I decided that I should invest in some quality running gear, so I went to a local running store and got fitted for shoes and inserts. When I told the salesperson that I was planning to run my first 5k, he said, "You'll be back here in a year because you'll want to run a 10k, and then in a couple years, you'll tell me you signed up for a half. Trust me; this sport is addicting". I laughed and said, "No way. I'm definitely stopping at a 5k". My sister and I ran that first 5k for our mother, who had recently been diagnosed with lung cancer.

Well, here it is, a little over two years later, and as you see from the picture above, I just ran my first half (notice I called it my first, because I know there will be others). I've battled shin splints, IT band issues, bronchial asthma—which ironically helped me to get my asthma under control through trying different treatments—and knee issues. But I've also made more new friends than I can count, lost most of those extra pounds I was carrying around, set a good example for my son, and, as several people have confessed, inspired them to step outside their comfort zones and try running. Half marathon training was one of the most physically demanding things I had undertaken, but I learned that I am capable of so much more than I thought in the process. To keep myself in the moment during the race and help make every moment count, I vowed that I would run each mile of my half for someone I loved, including my husband and son. I ran one mile for those who can't, including the victims of the Sandy Hook school shooting and the 9/11 attacks. I ran one mile for my departed friends and relatives. I ran one for my mother, who eventually succumbed to her illness, and one mile for the friends who've supported and encouraged me along my journey. I left one mile—the last mile—without a dedication; and that is because I ran that one for me. Every mile counts.

It has only been two years, but I have come so far and done so much good through running that I never want this journey to end. I may not win races or have a runner's physique, but I have the heart of a champion, and for as long as I can, I will make every step count and run with all I have.

Thank you
Michele Ridolfi O'Neill
10/14/15

Every Mile Matters
by Sarah L.A.C.E.

I have written and rewritten what I want to say over the last several months. Each month there is something different. A different angle to the same reason I run.

I grew up with some difficulties and in 2003 I was finally told my diagnosis of Borderline Personality Disorder. I spent much of my time prior to and after the diagnosis self-medicating. Then around 2009 I was asked if I wanted to be part of a running team for the Manitoba Marathon held every Father's Day. I agreed to it and then panicked. I hadn't run since high school and then it was only on track and field day, going for 100meters. But I did it and ran just over 3 miles for my leg of the race. Between the practice with the Couch to 5k and the race, I remembered why I loved to run. (If you ask my mom she'll say that I never did walk anywhere, I ran.)

An extra bonus was that it was providing me with the high my body was craving and helping me stay connected to myself by keeping my moods stable. And I got the control I needed to feel sane. I couldn't control anything about my life or the disorder, but I could control how far and long I ran for. For short spurts, I could control how fast I ran as well. And of course the medal at the end rocked. Crossing that finish line helped me feel accomplished with something I was doing in my life. (I currently have a team relay, a 5k, a 10k, 2 half marathons, a virtual 10k, and a color run under my running belt. I hope to run a full marathon when I'm 40 so I can say I did it.)

This past year I haven't been able to run as much. I got really sick with anxiety. Something that came up in high school but appeared to be a secondary symptom to the BPD. So essentially it was ignored. There was no ignoring it now. I was losing my life. I couldn't even go outside without getting sick. My favorite was running outdoors, so this was a cause of severe depression.

The last five months have been me getting better and healthier with the help of medication and therapy. So now I run because I can. I am healthy physically, I have my legs and I am blessed enough to be able to utilize my body to run. This is why every mile matters to me. Every mile means a healthier mood day for myself. To enjoy the great life God gave me. To enjoy my husband, children, family and friends. I am blessed, and each mile I run I am celebrating that I can.

Why Every Mile Matters, And Each Step Counts
By Laurie Winslow

The shoe set to pavement makes a shushing sound against the ground,
Steps shush the din of the past, encouraging the next step, and next.
Each heartbeat presses forward pumping hope through a tired soul.
Each breath in, pushing out the past, refreshing the mind, renewing.

The birds and squirrels watch me pass, and continue rushing about.
They do not care where my race began, or where it will end.
Moments earlier the office, the family, the friends, made me the same.
Each step leaves that frenzy in my past, each breath in, affords clarity.

Runners pass, and I pass others, the same path different for everyone.
Shoes accompanied by a cane, tapping defiance at the couch calling.
Each step a victory, when each start is half the struggle alone.
Steady, ready, step again, and leaving the past behind.

The road doesn't care if I wasn't good enough for the promotion
It doesn't care if my home is perfect, or what my social status is.
While the TV and couch wait, the road just listens, hearing calm.
The road is building a "Yes, you can", and "You are worth every mile"!

Laced my shoes because the doctor said I had to make a change,
That starting line can feel so cold and hard, ominous and waiting.
Finish lines along the way call me forward like many rustling leaves,
The cheering of chippering birds and chattering squirrels spur me on.

The road looks long, but carries me each step along over every mile.
The lungs clear, the body becomes more toned, the cane is left behind.
Tomorrow people line the street and others run beside me,
Pass the finish, and note my time, success! No longer impossible!